CONSEQUENCES of OPPRESSION
Pt. 2

Women in Danger

By PEN BLACK

A Serious Conversation for Women of Color

Goal: To help instruct Women of Color on how to better obtain Power, How to better maintain Power, and how to better utilize Power - while protecting yourself from other more pernicious uses of Power.

DEDICATION

I dedicate this book to all Women, especially Women of Color, Original women.
Your journey have been the longest, your struggles have been the hardest, end your triumphs have been the greatest.

I also give the deepest thanks to the two -women that supported me the most and have inspired me beyond measure
-my mother Renee Johnson and my sister Sherice Johnson, both who returned back to the essence far too soon.

THANKS

I want to give special thanks to: Syreeta Davis for being supportive in so many ways and to Ms. Diane for having her. Carol Blades for being the consummate friend; Keona Center for being the sister I needed; Barbara Abadia for being my Spanish connect; Faatma Behesht for sharing so much of her wisdom with me; Antika Truitt for being such a talented thinker and author Yafeesa Johnson for being my favorite survivor and writer.

And to all Women of Color, your beauty inspires me to do more!

Table of Contents

Part One

Part Two

INTRODUCTION

Peace,

I decided to talk to the women because there is no-one in the universe more precious to me. Women are by far God's most priceless jewel, and the fountain of joy that is all a man really needs to drink from for sustenance and fulfillment. That's why I am also appalled at the condition of our women today. How did we let our women suffer so much, lose so much, and have to deal with such misery? This conversation focuses more on Blackwomen, because of more dire need.

How did we let our refined, intelligent, strong, beautiful Blackwomen come to this? How could our original women, full of melanin, our sisters and mothers be 23 times more likely to have HIV or AIDS than a whitewoman. How could we let our perfectly created Blackwomen now become a population of nearly 60% overweight or obese?

I am so disappointed at the Blackman and the job he has done of protecting, providing for, loving, and guiding the Blackwoman. We just went thru a period of unparalleled prosperity and so what the Blackman drove big cars, made a lot of money, wore a bunch of fashions, and fucked a bunch of women. Look at what we let happen to our mothers our daughters, our sisters, and our wives - if we were man enough to marry them. How the hell did we let our women become the leaders of almost every negative category?

1. Most likely to have HIV or AIDS
2. Most likely to live in poverty
3. Most likely to drop out of high school
4. Most likely to be sexually abused
5. Most likely to be overweight or obese
6. Most likely to suffer domestic homicide
7. Most likely to be a teen-mom
8. Most likely to be a single mother
9. Most likely to have love ones in jail
10. Most likely to wind-up in jail
11. Most likely to die of a heart-attack
12. Most likely to have her men turn their backs on her.

When Does It End? When Do We Say Enough!

I propose that starting right now women stop waiting for men to stand-up and take responsibility for them. That women realize no duty is more important, more sacred than protecting themselves, their children, and then their men. These conditions were allowed to fester and grow, mostly because the men were too engaged in their own selfish, stupid, savage pursuits. Now our women are dying; physically, mentally, and spiritually - alone and in misery. It's about time we realize The Earth was made to be a paradise for a deserving man.

These are dire times, requiring a serious conversation, and a more focused attempt at securing real Power.

Empowering women starts with the attainment of Power and Power is not given freely, it is something that has to be taken.

The pursuit of Power is often looked at as an amoral pursuit, something that should only be actively sought by the wicked. Yet, when a force so strong, so influential, so pervasive is left in only the hands of the wicked, the rest of the world is subjected to the cruel, oppressive and tormenting atrocities that have so commonly plagued the human race.

I feel the only way for people and especially Black People to protect themselves from the whims of others is to obtain and wield their own high levels of Power.

The obtainment of Power is an arduous, often dangerous endeavor that lies outside the confines of the common rules, usually set in place to keep the powerless from ever changing their status.

This book is designed to help change a person's status, to wrestle Power away from others and hold on to it by 'Any Means Necessary.' This is not a good guy book or a bad guy book, but an 'I'm tired of not having enough control over my status in life' book. This book can help the weak become strong, the have-nots start having, and the powerless become Powerful.

In order to obtain Power, we must first understand what it is. Power is the often subtle, but always pervasive ability to influence, effect, change, or control; a person, a group, your environment, or the world around you. We have to regain that Power over ourselves, our environment, and our circumstances.

Most people are conditioned to view the pursuit of Power as an evil under-taking. It is convenient for the powerful to have the least powerful of people to think of Power as evil, or the pursuit of Power as wrong. Nobody likes powerlessness; everyone wants Power - even if they are too deceitful or naïve to admit it. Power takes place in every aspect of life - even between friends and lovers, brothers and sisters, child and parent, teacher and student, employer and employee, citizens and government, and mere acquaintances and strangers. There is no escaping the struggles for Power; it permeates every inch of our existence. In the struggle for Power, you can either be a victor —of which there are few, or a victim - which there are plenty. This book will help you choose one - and become that.

This book is not for the person just trying to get by, just survive, or just make it. This is the Women of Color much needed guide to obtain real Power; over themselves, and over their surroundings, in an oppressive society, and in the world at large.

To obtain real Power- will require strength, fortitude, sacrifice, and a ruthless pursuit of goals. Most important, to gain real Power requires a constant elevation of mind, money, or status.

To remain powerless will make you vulnerable at any time to misery, poverty, enslavement, and death! Remember, once you have real Power, you can do what you want - be who you want, even one of the nicest, most generous persons alive - if that's what you choose.

This book is about the obtainment of Power and remember, Power is never given freely - it must be taken; either by force, influence, coercion, or manipulation.

<u>WOMEN</u>

Women strive, triumph, survive,
suffer neglect from every side,
gallant smiles disguise their cries,
over and over I hear - God why ?

From Vanilla to Chocolate,
seems your struggles are the hardest, there's
strength in your darkness,
been that way since we started.

CHAPTER 1

Dying to Eat vs. Eating to Live

To obtain and maintain Power requires a person have plenty of energy to work harder and be smarter than most. Bad health and sickness is a barrier to people being at their optimum; besides the fact it would be a waste to gain great Power and be too ill to enjoy it.

We know the best knower of Us and our needs is Us. We now let the poison animal eaters, slave makers of the poor, and capitalist cannibals dictate to us what and how we should eat. We have the most well- crafted, most perfectly made, most divinely made physiques on Earth, now becoming the most over-weight, obese, sick, diseased and dying. 60% of Black people in America are over-weight and 34% are considered obese-We are suffering the most because Caucasian's ways are most ill-suited for our righteous physiology.

In this chapter I will challenge what we have been taught is the right way to eat. What we eat and how we eat is wrong, it is not designed for Original people, (Blackpeople), and it's killing Us. Once again we have been tricked into our own self-destruction to keep the food industry making trillions of dollars by shoveling an estimated 70 tons of food down each American's mouth. Those 70 tons are scientifically designed to keep you eating more and getting more sick so the medical industry who write over 4 billion prescriptions a year can continue making their trillions.

The first thing we need to know is that most diseases have one single cause and one single solution. The cause is that 70 tons of food you eat in a lifetime have over-burdened your Lymph System to the point it can no-longer rid the body of enough toxins or enough toxins fast enough. The solution is to clean your Lymph System and keep it clean and healthy so it can do its job, which is - Keep You Alive and Disease Free.

Of course most people don't know anything about The Lymph System and the Food Industry and Medical Industry wants to keep it that way. I want you to know all about your waste/toxin/disease fighting system, so you can all live long, healthy, disease free lives.

Every second of every day, the body accumulates toxic waste matter and must eliminate this toxic waste. Internally, hundreds of billions of cells are replaced every day. The old cells are toxic and must be eliminated by the eliminative organs; the bowels, the bladder, lungs and skin. We have no control of the internal waste production or its elimination. When the build-up of toxins exceeds what the body can naturally get rid of then you develop a clogged, backed-up, toxic-filled, self-poisoned body.

The single greatest contributor of toxic waste to our bodies is the 70 tons of food we eat during a lifetime. The chemical exposure we receive from our foods, dramatically increases the demands for nutrients to try and detoxify these multiple toxic concoctions. When food is eaten, it has to be broken down and separated into two parts: the energy and nutrients the body needs to survive, and all the toxic matter the body needs to rid itself of. When the accumulation of toxic elements becomes greater than The Lymph System's ability to discard toxins, the body develops Toxemia.

Toxemia is when more toxins are being produced in the body than The Lymph System can break down and eliminate. Disease, bad health and sickness are the point where the toxins have overwhelmed the body's ability to contain them. If not for Toxemia, there would be no Diabetes, Arteriosclerosis (heart Disease), Colitis, Appendicitis, Crohn's Disease, no Eczema, no Cancer... basically all diseases start with Toxemia.

The Lymph System's job is to collect garbage; it works 24 hours a day to keep the inside of the body clean and rejuvenated. The Lymph System is an amazing network of fluid, organs, nodes and nodules, ducts, glands, and vessels that continuously and aggressively cleanse the system of waste matter. Millions and millions of lymph nodes, some minute, some large, guard the various passages into the body against the intrusion of destructive substances. One such lymph gland visible in the mouth is the tonsil; which provides a protective ring of lymph tissue around the opening between the nasal and oral cavities. The tonsils protect against bacteria and other dangerous materials, if some misguided doctor doesn't convince you to snatch your tonsils out. The lymph vessels in the body would cover a distance of over 100,000 miles. They would circle the globe 4 times. The lymph fluid in your body is 3 times more than the amount of blood in your body; that's how important The Lymph System is unlike the circulatory blood system. The Lymph System carries fluid only away from the tissues. It picks up waste from all the cells through an intricate series of processes - break them down and arrange the elimination of them from the body. The Lymph System is also involved in the production of white blood cells (lymphocytes) that seek out, capture, and destroy foreign substances such as bacteria, toxins, and other haphazard materials, and remove them from the body.

When The Lymph System is so over-whelmed with toxins and waste material that it no-longer can do its job properly, we become sick, diseased, and start to die. The body is so perfectly engineered to take care of itself that, even when our destructive eating habits damage it, we get plenty of warning signs to 'Change'.

The seven most pronounced warning signs are:

1. Enervation - which is a condition where the body isn't generating enough energy to perform it's necessary tasks. The body becomes impaired and starts generating even less energy; including the processes of elimination of the toxic by-products of both metabolism and the residue of the 70 tons of food consumed by the body. You become tired and sluggish and require more sleep. Loss of Appetite is the biggest indicator that your body is in distress, because digestion requires a significant output of energy. When extra energy is needed to heal the body, natural wisdom and intelligence of the body send signals to not eat to free up that energy usually used for digestion. This is stage 1.

2. Toxemia - also referred to as toxicosis or autointoxication is when the un-eliminated toxic material in the body starts to saturate the blood, lymph nodes, and tissues of the body. The body recognizes Toxemia as a hazardous situation and attempts to flush out the toxins, when this happens, you can expect more physical discomfort and an even greater drain of the body's energy supply. It's also during this stage that a very obvious and necessary symptom occurs -fever. A fever mobilizes the body's defenses when there is an emergency. When there is an accumulation of toxins in the body, metabolism is accelerated by increasing the amount of heat available; which enhances the healing process. Metabolism consists of the absorption of nutrients and the elimination of wastes. Heat acts as a catalyst which causes the toxins to liquefy and pass into the bloodstream, where they are transported to the organs responsible for waste removal (bowels, bladder, lungs and skin) and out the body. Fever is part of the second stage and if toxemia isn't severely reduced, the next stage of disease develops.

3. Irritation – the body's nagging discomfort like itchiness, feeling queasy or nauseated, short-tempered, nervousness, depression, and anxiety could all be the body's way of getting your attention. Irritation is another of the body's warning signs, telling you your toxin level is too high. The irritation is usually not enough to see a doctor, but enough to go noticed. If enervation, toxemia, and irritation are ignored long enough, the fourth stage of disease ultimately takes place.

4. Inflammation - Is the body's most intense effort to cleanse itself and restore good health- When this stage occur, you are keenly aware because it involves pain. The body's most effective warning is pain. When pain is chronic and unrelenting, it is a sign that the body is desperately trying to rid itself of toxins before it causes more   damage.
With inflammation, the toxins have usually concentrated into a particular organ or particular area for a massive elimination effort-This area becomes inflamed because of the constant Irritation from the toxins. Many people at this juncture take medications to suppress the symptoms, and continue to ignore the cause. If left unchanged and toxins are not drastically reduced, the next stage of disease will begin. Stage 4 is a crucial time to make healthy change because right now the body is more than half-way towards a full blown disease.

5. Ulceration - This stage means the body has been under attack for a long time and cells and tissue are being destroyed. This condition is usually very painful because there are exposed nerves. Lesions and ulcers can occur on the inside of the body and on the outside. For example - a stomach ulcer is a hole in the stomach caused by to many toxins and is an inside ulcer. A canker sore on the mouth, or a oozing sore on the arm or leg are outside ulcers used as an outlet to rid the body of toxins. Ulcers will heal If toxemia levels are lowered, if not the next stage of disease begins.

6. Induration - Scarring is a form of induration. The hardening of tissue or the filling in of tissue where it was lost, like an ulcer, is the body's last ditch effort to encapsulate toxins. The toxins are trapped in a sack of hardened tissue, to quarantine the toxic material before it can spread to other parts of the body. The sac is a type of tumor and is very often diagnosed as cancer, even though no cancer is present. Induration is the last stage where the body is still in control of its cells. If the destructive habits that bought about these first 6 stages continue, cells go crazy, they become parasitic - living off the body's nutrients and contributing nothing in return. The constant toxic poisoning has altered the cells genetic coding and has caused them to become wild and disorganized - now you have a full blown disease.

7. Disease - such as cancer is now trying to destroy the body- At this point in the evolution of disease, if the cause of the earlier stages isn't arrested, bought under control - the results are usually fatal. The body vitality is at its lowest point and cells are no no-longer under the brain's control.

Even in disease the body strive to maintain a healthy state, because health is natural, illness is not. At this point, if a healthy lifestyle is adopted, corrective measures are taken to remove toxins, the disease will progress no further, and the body will heal. The body itself is the best healer; drugs can mask the symptoms while the toxin overload persists, and this progression usually ends in death.

That's how we are killing ourselves with an over-abundance of toxins, from the 70 tons of food we eat in a lifetime. Now I will tell you how to eat to live, so you can live a long life free of pain, illness, disease, and the medical industry's poison prescriptions.

First and foremost, it's okay to enjoy food, to enjoy eating, you should live abundantly - not in a constant state of worrying about your food intake. You should not suffer from hunger or feel deprived and most of all you should not experience loss of energy and health from your food. This is about eating as much as you want; the proper way so you can have a healthy, beautiful, vibrant body, full of energy and stamina.

The number 1 mistake people make with food is combining food items improperly. If we were to start right now combining our foods properly, we would have abundant energy, slim, healthy bodies, proper nutrients, beautiful skin, feel great and live longer - without sickness.

Food combining is based on the discovery that the digestion of food takes more energy than any other function in the body and certain combinations of food may be digested with greater ease and efficiency than others. The human body is not designed to digest more than one different type of concentrated food in the stomach at the same time. A concentrated food is any food that is not a fruit of a vegetable. Fruits and vegetables are not concentrated foods, they are High- Water Content foods. These High-Water Content foods are filled with natural water the body needs for nourishment and cleansing. All the vitamins, minerals, proteins, amino acids, enzymes, carbohydrates, and fatty acids the body needs - are to be found in fruits and vegetables. From a scientific and a common-sense standpoint; when you realize that our planet is 70 percent water, our bodies are 70 percent water, it makes perfect sense that our diet should be approximately 70 percent water content. That means fruits and vegetables should make up 70 percent of our diets and the other 30 percent should consist of the concentrated foods; breads, grains, meat, dairy product, legumes and so on.

Most people clean the outside of their body every day and the inside never. Then we wonder why our bodies are clogged, full of toxins, lacking energy, and nearly 60' percent of the people are over-weight. Water transport nutrients to all the body's cells and remove toxic waste. The water in fruits and vegetables carry the full nutritional requirements into the intestines, where all nutrients are absorbed. Regular water, vitamins and supplements can never replace the job of fruits and vegetables - which is to provide all the body's nutritional requirements while thoroughly, efficiently, and naturally cleaning the inside of our bodies.

Food digestion requires more energy than any other activity humans do; more than walking, swimming, or running. When foods are not properly combined, they sit in the stomach extra hours sapping energy and becoming rotten. For example: all meats and dairy are protein and the stomach recognizes proteins with an acid digestive juice.   All rice, breads, and pastas are starches and the stomach recognizes starches with an alkaline digestive juice.   Now what do you think happens when acid juice and alkaline juice is created in the stomach at the same time - they neutralize each other and the stomach keeps making more juice, wasting valuable time and energy trying to digest.   After as long as eight hours in the stomach, this improperly combined food is only partially digested. The protein has become putrefied and the starch has fermented, the nutrients cannot be incorporated into the healthy cells and more toxic waste is created. After hours and hours in the stomach, this rotten food is forced down the 30 feet of intestines, draining the body of energy and depriving the body of valuable nutrients.   Years and years of improper food combining creates these overweight, toxin-filled, nutrient deprived bodies lacking adequate energy and getting sick and dying young unnecessarily.

Most of the foods we eat clog our bodies, not clean them.   No other food is more delicious or nutritious for the body than fruit, but fruit needs to be eaten properly. Fruit is such a high-water content food that digestion is very quick and easy and requires the least amount of energy. To properly eat fruit, it needs to be alone or with only other fruit. Fruit is 80 to 90% cleansing, life-giving water, it creates no toxic waste and when eaten fresh and alone - it passes almost immediately from the stomach to intestines for absorption. When eaten with other foods or on a stomach not empty, it ferments and rots in the stomach and the body doesn't receive all its life-supporting essentials.   Fruit should be eaten alone, on an empty stomach, at least 20 minutes before any other foods.

Meats require the most energy to digest, they take twice as long as any other food to pass thru your gastrointestinal tract, and meats create the most toxins. Protein is more easily obtained at a much better quality, from fruits, vegetables, nuts and seeds. Meats drain our bodies of-enormous amounts of energy, live in our bodies rotting away for days, create the most toxins and lead to the most Illness. If one must consume meats it should be alone, the best quality, and very limited. You would be giving your body the best gift by reducing or eliminating meats.

Dairy products are the second most destructive food to your body -despite the lies we are taught our whole lives. The enzymes necessary to break down and digest milk are renin and lactase. By the age of three, most humans have very little renin and lactase to digest milk. All milk contains casein and cow's milk has three hundred times more casein than in human milk. Casein coagulates in the stomach, forming large, thick difficult to digest curds. Cows have a four – stomach digestion system equipped for casein. In humans casein turns into a thick mass of goo that is an enormous burden on the body and requires an extremely tiring amount of energy. That goo from milk hardens and sticks to the lining of the intestines, preventing the absorption of nutrients.

Milk creates large amounts of mucus that coat the mucus membranes and forces the whole body to perform sluggish. Vital energy is always wasted and weight loss become two to three times more difficult when the body is full of mucus. Dairy products have also been linked to heart disease, cancer, arthritis, migraine headaches, allergies, ear infections, colds, asthma and respiratory ailments.

If milk is consumed, it should be absolutely alone and on an empty stomach. Cheese is better alone or with a vegetable, and yellow cheese should be avoided since it's just heavily dyed cheese.

Most people believe milk and dairy products are necessary for calcium, when the truth is all green leafy vegetables and all raw nuts provide an abundance of calcium and a better quality -of calcium. The body uses calcium to neutralize acid. Dairy products actually causes the body to use calcium to neutralize it's acidic effects. That's why, even though Americans drink more milk and consume more dairy products than any other country, America also leads the world in Osteoporosis. Milk and its products have debilitating effects on the human body and isn't ideal for human consumption. Babies need breast milk and cow's milk is made for calves!

This Is How You Eat To Live and if you want to really help your body operate at optimum level, you should adhere to the body's natural cycles. The body has a natural time to eat, to absorb, and to eliminate.

Cycle 1 - Elimination (4a.m. - noon) is the time your body naturally works at elimination of toxic waste and food by-products. This is not the time to eat concentrated foods or a breakfast of anything other than natural fruit juice or fruits. Elimination is most critical to the cleaning of your body and eating anything other than fruit (which require least energy of all food to digest) halts the process to deal with new food and its toxic load. Elimination process not being interrupted is the most important time and activity needed for weight loss.

Cycle 2 -Appropriation (noon - 8 P.M.) This is the natural eating period. Concentrated foods, meals (properly combined of course), any stimulants like tea or coffee, and any kind of supplements should be taken now. This is the best time for your body to enjoy your food and make best use of its nutrients, because you are not interrupting its other cycles.

Cycle 3-Assimilation (8 P.M. - 4 A.M.) This is when the body gets a chance to extract, absorb, and utilize all the nutrients from the food you have eaten. No absorption of nutrients can take place until the food reaches the intestines, which takes about 3 hours for properly combined foods - about 8 hours for improper. It's best to eat your last meal at least 3 hours before you retire at night and early enough for the food to be totally assimilated before 4 A.M. and the start of the next cycle.

There you have it: An easy, comprehensive way to eat properly, cleanse the body, rid yourself of toxins, and stay healthy. Of course, this chapter was not intended to replace or interfere with existing medical treatment or advice, be smart - follow your doctor's advice, but nothing but good will come from allowing your own body to stay clean and healthy with a clean and healthy Lymph System that's not over-worked and over-whelmed.

This is not a diet; this is not meant to leave you hungry and deprived. You can eat just about as much as you want and whatever you want, and be healthy, slim, full of energy, and never go hungry -if you food combine properly and make fruits and vegetables the majority of your food intake. If you eat meats and dairy, just be mindful of how you eat it and how much, because they require the most energy to digest and create the most toxins. Of course, for the very best you, a little exercise goes a long way - even 20 minutes of walking a day will increase your health and longevity. Remember, it's not being over-weight that makes you sick, but the unhealthy eating habits that made you overweight, that makes you sick.

I hope this chapter will help you live a long, healthy, happy life, full of abundance and vitality. The two biggest health threats to Blacks in America is heart disease; specifically Atherosclerosis. The other is HIV and AIDS. This chapter can help prevent and possibly cure the first, but a hell of a lot more has to be done to stop the epidemic spread of HIV and AIDS. Let's Start!

The Invisible Enemy:
Atherosclerosis

Atherosclerosis is the 'hardening of the arteries'. This disease is the cause of chest pain, heart attack, and stroke. No-one is immune to this disease but healthy habits can slow its progression and prevent its development Atherosclerosis develops slowly over time. Studies have shown plaque buildup in the arteries starts in childhood, and fatty streaks have been found in teenager's arteries. Smoking, high blood pressure, high cholesterol, diabetes, advancing age, and even a high fat meal damages your endothelium; the smooth inner layer of cells that line healthy arteries and regulate blood flow. Bad habits, unhealthy conditions, and becoming older cause arteries to become stiffer and less responsive. Over time, the endothelium becomes so damaged and scarred that it is unable to completely repair itself and plaque starts to buildup.

The heart is usually the first place to show symptoms of Atherosclerosis, because of its constant workload and need for blood. When it manifests itself as chest pain or angina during exertion, Atherosclerosis is called Coronary Artery Disease. No matter where the symptoms manifest, Atherosclerosis is a condition that affects the whole body.

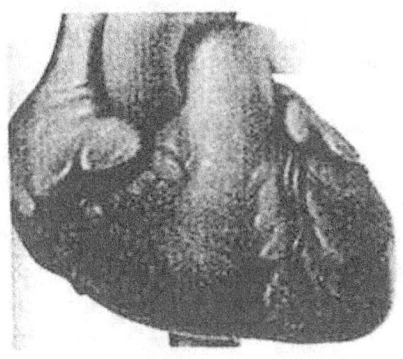

If plaque buildup and stiffening of the arteries is found in one part of your body, then it is present everywhere in the body. In different parts of the body the symptoms and damage are different, but Atherosclerosis is still the culprit. When atherosclerosis causes blocked arteries in the arms and legs, it is called Peripheral Arterial Disease. Kidney failure can occur when plaque buildup in the renal arteries. When the carotid arteries, which are the main blood vessels to the brain becomes blocked by plaque – this is called Cerebrovascular Disease. Atherosclerosis is even the culprit in many cases of erectile dysfunction.

If plaque buildup cause a rupture, a crack, or a clot big enough to block the flow of blood in the artery; organs and tissue downstream can be damaged or die due to lack of blood and oxygen. If blood flow is interrupted in an artery - this becomes a heart attack. If blood flow is interrupted in the carotid artery or brain - this becomes a stroke. Atherosclerosis can also cause an aneurysm - which is the bulging or ballooning of the artery.   If an aneurysm suddenly ruptures, uncontrolled bleeding can develop and lead to death.

Everyone is at risk, but no-one has to develop life-threatening conditions of Atherosclerosis. Even though advancing age and heredity contribute to Atherosclerosis, a life-long process of behavior, habits, and risk factors are the biggest determinates.

It is never too early to start making healthy living choices to prevent or minimize Atherosclerosis. Smoking and second hand smoke does extensive damage to your endothelium. Smoke makes blood platelets stickier, raise heart rate and blood pressure and increases the onset of Atherosclerosis and it's damage to the body.

Regular exercise helps control the blood pressure, cholesterol, weight gain, and it helps keep the artery walls flexible. A diet low in saturated fats, full of fruits and vegetables, whole grains, and monosaturated fats limit artery damage.

If you have risk factors like; diabetes, high blood pressure, or high cholesterol, make sure you get screened regularly for Atherosclerosis.

Affected site	Complication

Cerebral arteries (brain) ········· Stroke, TIA (mini stroke)

Carotid arteries (neck) ········· Stroke, TIA (mini stroke)

Aorta (heart) ········· Aneurysm

Coronary arteries (heart) ········· Angina (chest pain), heart attack

Renal arteries (kidneys) ········· Hypertension, kidney failure

Iliac arteries ········· Peripheral arterial disease

Femoral arteries

Tibial arteries

20

Millions Battle PAD

Peripheral arterial disease occurs when narrowed arteries reduce blood flow to your extremities, mostly your legs and pelvis. Many people who have been diagnosed with atherosclerosis also have PAD.

Most people realize they have it after experiencing painful cramps in their hips, thighs, or calves when walking or exercising. Early diagnosis and treatment is key to help prevent further damage.

Chapter 2

Death by Sex!

HIV and AIDS is the greatest threat we Original People (Blackpeople) may have ever faced. Right now Blackwomen are the casualty of war; soldiers without a helmet, without a weapon, and without much ground support. Do you know that nearly 70% of all new HIV and AIDS reported are Blackwomen? Do you know Blackwomen are now 23 times more likely to have HIV or AIDS than a whitewoman? Did you know that men (your Blackmen) are spreading HIV and AIDS to you women more than 10 times as fast as women spread it-Yes! He is willing to kill you for 20 minutes of pleasure, and about 80% of the time you aren't getting a husband, not getting a father for your children- and not even getting a long-term loving relationship out the deal. Damn! I mourn your circumstances, but don't let them mourn you! Wrap-up, get him and yourself tested, or be celibate, or get a toy, are at the very least Be More Serious, Selective- and Self-Aware! No dick is worth dying for - I love pussy, but none is worth dying for! Our single most reliable protection, other than celibacy is condoms. Condoms are great, now they have all kinds of varieties. They have textured, bumpy surfaces, ticklers, and attachments that can vibrate. Condoms can be infinitely more interesting and exciting than skin and safe - So Use Them! Stop dying, stop getting sick, stop letting those irresponsible, ignorant brothers risk your life and the future of our families, communities, and Nation.

No-longer can you women let him dominate you in the bedroom, no-longer can you let him determine how and when to protect yourself. You are strong in everything else - be strong in sex. Now is the time to 'Just Do It', make him wear a condom - every time. Be a 'Survivor' or be a 'Independent Woman', with toys if necessary, but no more can you be 70% of the new HIV and AIDS, no more can you be 23 times more likely to have HIV or AIDS than a whitewoman, and no more can we sit back and let Black teenagers have 68% of all the teenage HIV and AIDS, when we as a people are only 12% of the American population. Damn! it's like HIV and AIDS is our middle name or something, and it's the greatest, least talked about epidemic ever - because It's Ours!

Who is infecting Who?   According to this article written by Vibe Magazine, it is Blackmen that are infecting Blackwornen - ten times as fast.

AIDS is spreading more quickly among women than among men now. The portion of female AIDS cases has grown from 7% in 1985 to 18% in 1994. Since 1981, more than 77% of those cases occurred among African-American and Hispanic women. In 13 U.S. Cities, AIDS is now the leading killer among women ages 25 to 44.

In October 1992, following a four-year public campaign by AIDS activists, added was gynecological conditions to its list of markers for the presence of HIV-the virus. The total number of AIDS cases rose 58% within two months, largely because cases were being counted differently. Women had been dying without ever knowing that they had AIDS.

Another reason that the number of women with AIDS is growing so rapidly is that men transmit the virus to women 10 times more often than the other way around. At N.Y. City's St. Clares Hospital, since 1981 they have monitored 18,217 cases in heterosexual women—double that of cases in heterosexual men (9,063).

Just as there are vastly different manifestations of AIDS between men and women, counselors say that the psychological impact is different for women too. 'Even if she's sick, a woman is usually going to take care of the household and the children first, and put herself last.'

This is part of the explanation for statistics showing that women dying of AIDS tend to die five or six times faster than men after being diagnosed. It's often the case that women are diagnosed later and at that point, the disease is more advanced.

FOR A WOMAN IS THERE ANYTHING MORE DANGEROUS THAN AN UNPROTECTED, IRRESPONSIBLE BLACKMAN WITH A DIRTY DICK?

How can we sustain any kind of Power if we don't protect our children? How can the future be brighter if we sit back and watch our children needlessly die premature, sickening deaths - almost before they are even mentally aware of all their promise and potential?

I am talking directly to you women because I know you care and unfortunately for Us as a people - it is you-women who are vastly alone raising our children. HIV and AIDS is running rampant through our communities and our children are standing right in its path. The latest 2009 Center for Disease Control report said that teenagers are the fastest growing group of people acquiring HIV and AIDS. Of that rapidly growing group of HIV and AIDS victims, 68% of them are African-American. Yes! Our children, Black teenagers have enormously higher numbers than all the other teenagers combined! We are dying fast, we are dying hard, and we are dying horrendously. Teenage HIV and AIDS is further decimating homes, communities, and our future Black Nation. Before we can work on solutions, we have to first get our heads out the sand, open our eyes wide and realize our children are hurting, lost and looking for guidance. In the meantime our teens are gambling with their lives - trying to find love, support, acceptance and excitement.

1 in 10 Black Teenage Girls Tested HIV-positive in D.C.

Washington, D.C, has one of the highest AIDS rates in the country; yet, fewer of those who are infected are seeking treatment, according to the advocacy group Metro TeenAIDS. Nationally, young African Americans were disproportionately affected by HIV infection, accounting for 55% of all HIV infections reported among persons ages 13-24 in 2004, notes the Centers for Disease Control and Prevention. Overall, more infections occurred in 2006 among people under age 30 than any other group, the CDC reports.

New HIV Infections in 2006   Estimated total: 54,300

Age 13-29 34%
Age 30-39 31%
Age 40-49 25%
Age 50+   10%

SOURCE: CENTERS FOR DISEASE CONTROL AND PREVENTION FACT SHEET, AUGUST 2008

DAMN! To other races we must look like the biggest cowards and losers. Sure, we helped a Blackman get elected President, but we can't or won't protect our little girls.

Where's the outrage? Where are the rallies and the marches? Where the hell is the media attention? Surely, the death and dying of Black Teenage Girls deserve as much attention as Rihanna and Chris Brown, Michael Jackson, and Tiger Woods -Right?

No- Wonder so many teenagers don't seem to care about nothing - We don't seem to care about them!

These numbers are terrifying; our children are sick, they are dying, and they are spreading HIV and AIDS at a breathtaking rate. How long before it reach one of our teens?

1 out of 10 Black Teenage Girls tested HIV Positive. That's an almost insanely high number with all the information about HIV and AIDS and all the ways to protect one's self available.

1 out of 10 means in a crowded classroom 3 of the girls probably have HIV. In a club as many as 40 girls are dancing, flirting, hooking up, have HIV and AIDS. On any street there could be about 4 or 5 HIV teenage girls running around. No-way we can ignore this! If we won't even care for our children, protect our children - then we might as well throw the towel in as a race. The children are our future and if 1 out of 10 is infected and still spreading to others - how long before half are infected and still spreading to others?

In 2009 teenagers were the fastest growing group testing positive for HIV and AIDS. Out of the whole population of teenagers, which Blacks only represent about 12%, Black Teenagers have 68% of the HIV and AIDS. With Black Teenagers being 68% and Blackwomen being approximately 70% of the newly diagnosed HIV and AIDS - How can we survive? Never have an epidemic been so wide spread and affecting a group of people so dis-proportionate and been so ignored by the Power Elite. That's why we have to become our own Power Elite. We need to get our own doctors healing us, psychologists warning us, and media broadcasting this to our children's ears and minds. This epidemic should be talked about every day, from every end of the world - until we have complete awareness, prevention, treatment, and a possible cure.

Why are we so overwhelmingly infected? Because we are waiting for others to solve our epidemic, instead of gathering our Power, gaining more Power, and using our Power to Save Ourselves.

HIV/AIDS in BLACK AMERICA

These statistics are so sobering; nobody should want to be in a party mood right now.

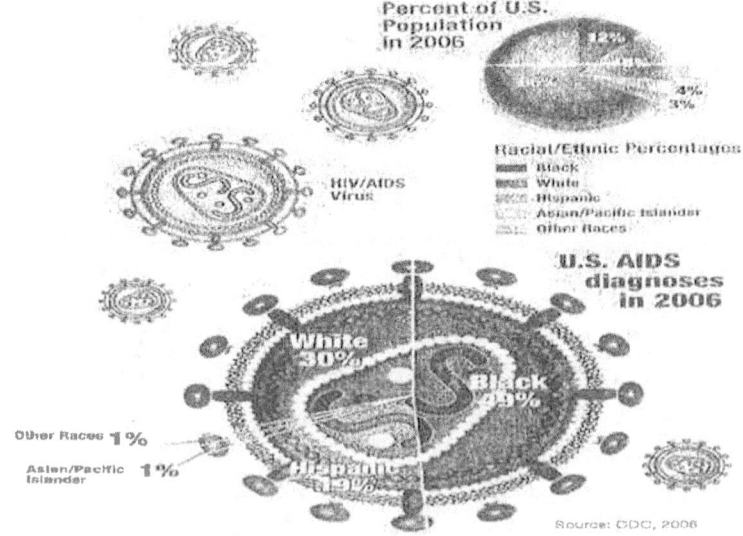

Source: CDC, 2006

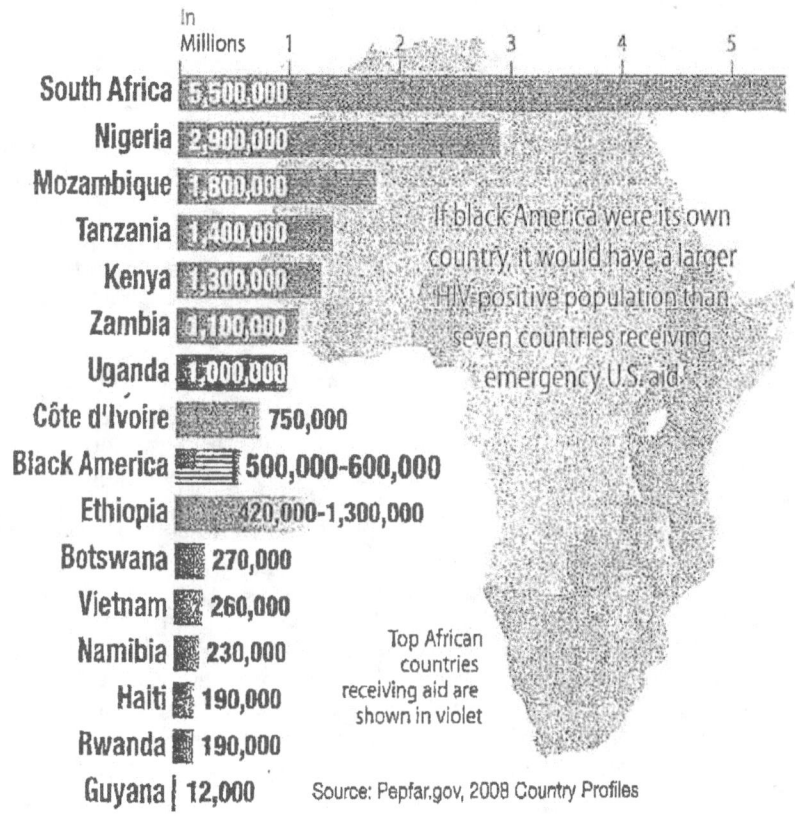

In Millions	1	2	3	4	5

South Africa 5,500,000
Nigeria 2,900,000
Mozambique 1,800,000
Tanzania 1,400,000
Kenya 1,300,000
Zambia 1,100,000
Uganda 1,000,000
Côte d'Ivoire 750,000
Black America 500,000-600,000
Ethiopia 420,000-1,300,000
Botswana 270,000
Vietnam 260,000
Namibia 230,000
Haiti 190,000
Rwanda 190,000
Guyana 12,000

If black America were its own country, it would have a larger HIV positive population than seven countries receiving emergency U.S. aid

Top African countries receiving aid are shown in violet

Source: Pepfar.gov, 2008 Country Profiles

Blacks represent 1 out of 8 Americans and 1 out of 2 persons with HIV and AIDS. If Black America were its own country, it would be the 35th most populous, with the 16th largest population of HIV and AIDS in the world.

AIDS remains the leading cause of death among Blackwomen between 25 -34 years old and the second leading cause of death in Blackmen between 35-44 years of age.

America spends billions of dollars combating HIV and AIDS around the globe, while virtually ignoring the epidemic here in Black America.

We better start saving our own ass, because nobody is gonna do it for us.

This is heart-breaking! Around the country half of all Black Teenage Girls are arriving at the doors of clinics, hospital, and morgues, more than at the door of colleges.

Now 68% of teenage HIV and AIDS belong to Black Teenagers in America, and these numbers are steadily climbing. Teenage HIV and AIDS is a wildfire raging out of control, that few are talking about and even less are doing something about.

We need some drastic measures - now! We need more awareness and a strong dose of reality presented to our youth. We need more infected teens and adults going to our schools and talking to our teens. We need doctors and patients in our churches and in the media bringing awareness. We need our popular rappers and entertainers bringing awareness to their fans. I feel scared straight programs are necessary; where school trips are arranged to hospitals and morgues so the teenagers can see the end results of unprotected sex. There should be incentive programs for getting tested and harsher punishment (community enforced) for infected individuals intentionally spreading the virus to others. We especially need our parents to open their eyes and heart to this epidemic and provide safe, stable environments for their children to talk, reveal their actions, even come to for sexual protection; like condoms and advice. We need condoms to be accessible and free, so that those who can't be persuaded to wait before becoming sexually active will at least have condoms readily available and obtainable. Schools, churches, community centers, even neighborhood eateries should have free condoms if necessary - whatever we have to do to protect our children. We have to attack the problem like it's a war for the lives of our children - Because It Is!

This article describes how HIV / AIDS can spread so rapidly.

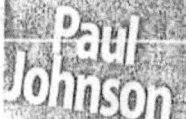

SEX WITH STRANGERS

From a man's perspective, you would have to be crazy not to love that gushy-ushy. Especially the way friction gives way to comfort, the way that sticky juice goes from sweet resistance to joyful slide. You have to love the way those walls clutch and grasp, pulsate and expand, engulf and exhale. What prize is more precious than hearing her ask for more? What sight is more beautiful than seeing her sweat flatten her hair, dance on her nipples, run between her breasts, cover her mid-section, and soak her hairs? Sex is why we dress the best, talk the slickest, hustle the hardest, and chase our prey like big-game hunters.

For me, new moans at night and fresh bellos in the morning is an almost unresistable enticement. So I understand promiscuity, I understand the triumph of winning the affection of multitudes of females. That new, unexplored territory, that first glimpse, that first kiss, that first touch, that first taste, and that first exhaustion. It often feels worth anything - but it's not! Unless she was a virgin when you met her and has remained totally monogamous - you are having sex with strangers.

Did you know that a recent report from the Centers for Disease Control and Prevention (CDC) indicates that 48% of African-American girls age 14-19 have a sexually transmitted disease. Funny how it's appeal when you think of a STD don't it? That sticky-icky can be sticky-sickly. She could be innocent enough to sell Girl Scout cookies,

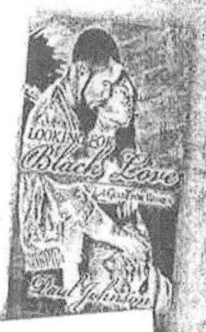

sweet enough to cry kool-aid, and fine enough to stop rush hour traffic. Can you really bet your life that every person she slept with, and every person they slept with was completely healthy? If she slept with just seven people that slept with seven people, that would be 57 people you are now sleeping with. With 48% of African-American girls with STD's and 70% of all newly diagnosed HIV - positive patients being African-American women, can you really afford not to wrap-up? I assume any men cool enough to be reading this superb magazine probably does pretty well with the ladies. So if you slept with atleast seven similar situations, you have given 56% strangers a good chance to get you sick or even take your life. Wrap-up if you want to live and enjoy that wet and wonderful tropical garden. Women are the world's most sensational creation and sex is our most joyful activity, but we can't risk our lives for it. Stop having unprotected sex with strangers before it's to late. Live long and healthy lives, and look-out next time you have sex with strangers

By Paul Johnson
Author of " A Lovely Murder DownSouth "
and " Looking For Black Love: Relationship Guide
For Women "

We as a people are too proud and valiant to just sit back and allow this man-made disease created to decimate our numbers and disturb our growth and development, to continue to kill and cripple us. It is time for us to fight back; in the day, in the night, behind closed doors, and in the media. It's time we fight harder for our own survival and the survival of our children. Maybe you need to be awakened, enraged, feel the indignation of what is really going on. We as a people were targeted for this disease and we have masterfully fallen victim to their devious plan: We are now the #1 contributor to our own self-destruction; Death by Sex!

Here's a quick history lesson, so you know it is no accident that a 12% population is 49% infected. That our women are 23 times more likely to be infected than a whitewoman. That our children are 68% of all the infected teens in America.

First of all, there is not and never was a Green Monkey that gave HIV or AIDS to Africans who later gave it to homosexuals, or that it started in Haiti. These groups; Africans, Haitians, and homosexuals were first blamed so this disease would be mostly ignored and over-looked by the general masses. According to extensive research and many leading authorities; such as Dr. Robert Strecker, a Los Angeles physician, Gastroenterologist and trained Pathologist; AIDS is a man-made disease created by splicing together Visna (sheep) and Bovine (cow) viruses, to make the human retro virus AIDS. The origin of AIDS has been traced back to a laboratory in Dietrich, Maryland. The virus was first spread by the World Health Organization in their Smallpox Vaccine, this was first reported by the London Times in a front page article titled "Smallpox Vaccine Triggered Aids Virus." The World Health Organization Smallpox Vaccine Program was during the early 70's and was in Brazil, Haiti, and Central Africa, where millions of Africans were inoculated.

In November, 1978 a Hepatitis B vaccine trial began on 1,083 white homosexual men (average age 29) in New York. In January of 1979 - a mere 2 months later, the first case of AIDS appeared in a homosexual in New York. In March 1980, an additional 1,402 gay men were vaccinated in five more cities; Chicago, Los Angeles, San Francisco, Denver, and St. Louis. Seven months later gay men had AIDS in Los Angeles and San Francisco.

HIV and AIDS were a deliberate, devised plan for 'Population Control' and Original People (Black People) were and still is its number 1 target. Research and see for yourself, but right now our number 1 task is to stop the spread of HIV and AIDS and stop the destruction of Blacks; especially our women and children. I say we stop financially supporting those that don't support our fight against this epidemic; starting with celebrities, businesses, media outlets, and politicians. If you are not part of the solution than you are part of the problem. Nothing is more important than our continued survival, if we don't start now taking more aggressive, pro-active steps to stop the bourgeoning flow of this epidemic, we as a race will look back in sorrow and ask, 'what happened to our best and brightest for the future?'

Chapter 3

No More Rape

Rape is the biggest theft of Power; it is debilitating and long-lasting. For thousands of years men have used rape to rob an individual of their strength, their security, and their sense of self-worth. All through history and current times, rape and sexual abuse has persisted, and women have overwhelmingly been its victim.

Rape is an inhumane crime that's not just perpetrated against the individual victim, but it is also a disruptive and destructive atrocity inflicted on societal and familial norms.

As stated by Naim Akbar, Ph.D. in "Breaking the Chains of Psychological Slavery":
> 'Families were broken up at the whim of the slave master. In addition, Blackmen were forced to watch their wives, daughters, sisters and mothers raped by their owners. Such experiences effectively disrupted the sense of connection and reciprocal protection that exists in the preservation of family systems. By undermining this loyalty and protective image for almost twenty generations or 400 years, one is able to create a painful alienation between men and women which continues to contaminate the reciprocal respect that men and women must have for each other in order to develop and maintain families.'

Rape was and is a physical and psychological weapon used to damage the souls of women and destroy the hearts of families.

In "Cultural Genocide" by Yosef ben-Jochannan, he states that:

'Rape of Blackwomen in America began 1619 or 1620 CE. when they first arrived in the Thirteen British Colonies that became the United States of America; before that the slave ships that bought them to the entire " Western World " -from ca. 1506; and even before that, as they walked up the gang plank to board the slave ships, but worst of all, they were raped in the presence of their Black ("negro male") Husbands, who were bounded with hands and feet tied to neck and testicles.'

Now, Blackmen not only witness the rape of Blackwomen - without the restraints of bondage to hold them back, but also actively, aggressively, and abundantly participate in the rape of Blackwomen; here in America, across the Caribbean, and deep in the bosom of Africa. All through the annals of time Whitemen have tried to use rape to demoralize and dehumanize Blackwomen. How much worst it is when Blackwomen own men treat her in similar ways.

A big silence has always blanketed the Black Community concerning the issues of rape, incest and sexual abuse. That silence is starting to be broken in a few movies, books and by some celebrities, but still very little is being done to protect our women and our youths. Plus, the attitudes of Black Males towards females are getting worst every day. Weak Black Males are using our women as sexual punching bags and age barely matters. Just a few days ago, I had to chastise a male old enough to have granddaughters, for making sexual advances towards an adolescent Black Female. He stated to me, "If she's old enough to bleed, she's old enough to be slaughtered." It took all my will-power to not knock more of his teeth out of his mouth, and his attitude is predominant among the Black Males in the hood, in the jails, and in our schools. Miserable hate-filled, misogynist males are lurking on our streets, our playgrounds, our schools, our work-place, and our homes. Most women and girls; especially our girls, are raped or sexually abused by someone very familiar to them. Sometimes it's a friend of the family, a neighbor, or casual acquaintance, but too often it's a daddy, step-daddy, uncle, or even a brother. That is one of the most devastating and destructive abuse of power and trust, when someone close to you rapes or abuses you. That theft of power, security and self-esteem lives inside a female forever, often causing a self-loathing that clouds her judgment and decision making. Treated like meat, feeling unprotected and unloved, many women engage in self-destructive, risky behavior. Many never see their full potentials as persons, repeatedly finding themselves in non-productive relationships. These women are even more likely to raise daughters that will suffer some kind of abuse. All this because we didn't protect our women, didn't protect our children, because we let these weak males get away with their misogynist thinking and their savage ways and actions. Like the way we let the R. Kellys' have sex with underage girls and for so long said nothing, did nothing. I wonder how many so-called men knew R. Kelly was preying on young girls and ignored it? I wonder how many of them said, "If she's old enough to bleed, she's old enough to be slaughtered."

I recently read the book "Push" by Sapphire and by page 23 I knew it was one of the best and worst books I ever read. I keep asking myself 'Are we really that bad? Can we really be that horrific, especially to children?' And I knew the answer was Yes! Some of us are that bad and worst.

In "Push", Precious is being raped by her own father and it starts in a bed with the mother awake, laying right beside them. Precious is raped from the age of 3 until she's 14, has two children by her father and nobody comes to her aid, not neighbors, not family, not school administration, not even welfare or social services after telling staff at hospital after birth of her first child - her father got her pregnant. Precious is also sexually, physically, and mentally abused by her mother on a daily basis. "Push" by Sapphire is a fiction based on facts, the book and movie resonates so loud, because it's circumstances are so real for millions of women and young girls every day. I am so glad the movie "Precious" based on the book "Push" by Sapphire is such an enormous success and I hope every person sees it, especially males, boys, and men - so they can all gain a greater sensitivity and humanity towards women and girls.

Another book that highlights the horrific conditions our young girls face is "A Lovely Murder DownSouth" by Paul Johnson. This fictional story is about a girl name Lovely who's being raped by her mother's boyfriends. Lovely is to paralyzed by fear to report the rapes and her mother is too afraid of losing her man to really look .at what's going on. Eventually Lovely's continued rape by men and neglect by her mother turns into a self-loathing. When Lovely grows up and get together with 2 other young women with their own reasons to hate men - Blackmen that remind them of their past abusers, the 3 ladies become the predators. Author Paul Johnson says "A Lovely Murder DownSouth" was written to try and show men how their negative, destructive, and sometimes monstrous treatment towards women do shape the actions of women for a lifetime; sometimes even turning prey into predator.

A recent study and survey was done on prostitution around the United States. In our Nation's capital, a few blocks away from our Black President, were streets full of prostitutes. Almost all of these street-walking DC prostitutes were Blackwomen with shockingly similar backgrounds. 75% of the prostitutes had been sexually abused and raped growing up; most of them raped by a trusted family member. 85% of these prostitutes were now addicted to heavy drugs. Plus, prostitutes have a 40% higher mortality rate than other DC residents; who already have one of the highest mortality rates in the country. Yes! because we don't protect our little girls when they are growing up they are much more likely to be sexually, physically and mentally abused as adults, be prostitutes, be addicted to drugs, and die early violent deaths. This is some of our best, our brightest turning to drugs, prostitution, dying premature deaths from AIDS and violence because we didn't protect them, didn't protect their innocence growing up.

Not even our women in the military are safe. Recent reports by Amnesty International show that women in the military are regularly being sexually abused and raped by the very comrades-in-arms they fight alongside. Most of the sexual assaults and rapes are done with impunity, because the military has a long-standing record for supporting a boy's club mentality that objectifies women and offer them little support.

Women in the military are subjected to even more sexual assaults and rapes while in combat zones; especially in Iraq and the Middle East. These women soldiers that do complain to military are often ignored, trivialized, or further victimized by reprisals in an unsympathetic atmosphere where the higher ups dismiss their complaints. These victims of 'military rape' eventually leave the service with a myriad of problems, including: various medical problems such as migraines, depression, panic attacks, and gynecological problems.

These women wind-up on many medications and while in the military, most never received adequate counseling for trauma or proper testing for sexually transmitted diseases.

According to Department of Defense statistics, the following figures offer dismal proof that even in the military our women aren't protected:

-74 - 85 percent of soldiers convicted of rape or sexual assault leave the military with honorable discharges (meaning rape conviction doesn't appear on their record).

-Only 2-3 percent of soldiers accused of rape are ever court marshaled.

-Only 5-6 percent of soldiers accused of domestic abuse are ever court marshaled.

This means our women aren't being all they can be, they are being robbed of their power and so much more, and we as a people are being robbed of their very best.

Sexual assault, rape, and incest are crippling, debilitating monstrosities inflicted on our young and innocent robbing them of physical, mental, and emotional power and we are not doing enough to stop it.

In Africa, conditions are even worse for women and children. Rape has always been a brutal consequence of war, but according to a recent report by Amnesty International, Rape and Sexual Assault are used as a deliberate military strategy, "an orchestrated combat tool." In Africa, rape is used to enforce terror, authority, and power over a person, group, or community.

In a segment of '60 Minutes' with Anderson Cooper, called "War Against Women: The Use of Rape as a Weapon in Congo's Civil War", it was reported that in the last ten years in the Congo, hundreds of thousands of women have been raped, most of them by male gangs.

What differs from rapes during wars of the past is - these aren't just soldiers bored reaping the so-called 'spoils of war', this is systematic destruction. Each battle is followed by pillaging, rape, and the terrorizing of villages. The women and girls are raped in the most brutal ways; often in front of husbands, family, and community to inflict terror and authority over that community. When these women are raped, it's the families and culture that's destroyed, since many of these societies view the women as repositories of a community's cultural and spiritual values. Even women that flee to so-called protected camps are raped there every single day. These women have to deal with physical damage, emotional injuries, and psychological torment. These women are ostracized by family and society, and many have contracted diseases. Far too often these women would rather commit suicide than live with the shame and pain.

In Darfur, the Janjaweed, an Arab militia aligned with the Sudanese government, uses rape as a weapon to ethnically cleanse Darfur and Eastern Chad of Blacks. Women and girls are brutally raped in front of husbands, family, and community to shame the women. Then the rapist cut the arms or other parts of the body to mark the victims as being raped and unsuitable as brides and compromised as mothers and wives.

A young girl reported to Amnesty International that; she and other girls were taken away by soldiers and forced to walk three hours to the military camp. At the camp they were beaten and told, "You the Blackwomen, we will exterminate you, you have no god." At night they were raped several times, she said, "The Arabs guarded Us with arms and we were not given food for three days."

Whether it's over in Africa, or here in America, rape is not a crime of passion, or just an isolated incident.

Rape and sexual assault is the biggest threat to Power you women face. You must protect yourselves and your children. Watch over your daughters even better than you watch your money. Watch the men around you and your children - all men, including family and especially your sex partners. Watch for any change in your child's behavior or avoidance of particular people - and take any signs, suggestions or alterations in behavior serious. When help is needed, seek' out organizations designed to help victims, get authorities involved, get love ones involved, move, buy protection; do what you have to do to protect yourself and your children.

Rape and sexual assault is a crime that handicaps your ability to climb, to soar, to reach your greatest heights - but it don't have to be, it can be used to become stronger and more determined to never be totally at the mercy of another person's power again. Rape can freeze a women's progress with fear and can last a lifetime - everyday robbing you of your Power to be your very best physically, mentally, and emotionally. If you are a victim, seek help, seek counseling, or find peer groups to help you work through the emotional residue.

Rape, sexual assault, incest and all types of sexual abuse can no-longer remain in the dark. We need to talk about it, admit it's going on far too much in our community and homes. We need to confront the silence and these insensitive monsters. We have to help those already affected by it and still going through it, overcome it's crippling effects and retain their Power and security so they can move forward and have happy, successful lives full of accomplishment and self-empowerment.

Protecting our women and children has to be our number one priority - Now
For those already affected by the above atrocities, let that anger, pain and dis-trust propel you to be smarter, stronger, and more ambitious about success and Power. Triumph over adversity is the best revenge and the best way to protect yourself in the future, so there can be **No More Rape!**

Chapter 4

Children

In the pursuit of excellence and prosperity, it is almost imperative that you put-off having children until you are firmly established in your path to Power. Children are a tremendous blessing, but they are also an extreme expenditure of time, energy, finances, and resources. Rare is the woman that can overcome the strain and strife of being a teenage mom, especially single, and still rise to the higher echelon of society and Power.

I am not saying don't have children; having children is a great thing. We need more intelligent, creative, unbounded, positive youths leading Us into tomorrow. What we don't need is more single young mothers and teen moms engaged in this constant battle for survival at the barest level. Too often early parenting becomes this joyous burden that deprives a young lady of continuing her education, pursuing her dreams, and accomplishing her goals. What happens is these strong and loving mothers, trade in a lot of their potential greatness for the care and development of their children. To sacrifice for their children shows their endless inner beauty. To protect yourself in your early years and have children when circumstances are more ideal, shows your inner intelligence.

Our children are better served when we parents bring them into a situation where there are two parents who are mentally, emotionally, and financially mature.

It is no accident that almost all of the most powerful and successful Blackwomen in America waited to have children or still haven't had any. People like Oprah, Tyra Banks, Beyonce, Venus and Serena are waiting. Others like astronaut Mae Jamison, Surgeon General - Dr. Joyce Elders, also prominent Latinas like Jennifer Lopez and Supreme Court Judge Sotomayor; TV producer - Mara Brock Akil, movie director - Julie Dash, politician -Maxine Waters, and lawyer, First Lady Michelle Obama, all waited to have children. Had these women been teen moms, or young single mothers, it is unlikely they would have been able to focus the time, energy, and resources needed to be as huge a success as they are. Even Michelle Obama, who has two incredible daughters waited till she had an established career and an established marriage before having children.

Ladies to acquire real Power requires intelligent planning, capitalizing on your strengths and resources, and years of focused, effective work. The early years, between 16 - 24 are usually the career building years and the 'Path to Power' will be smoother and more surmountable if parenting is put-off to after the early" developmental years for a young woman and her road to success.

Chapter 5

Education

In American society, the one great denominator that allows a person to excel and elevate to the heights of accomplishment despite their background is education. Any person can go from poverty to well-off through hard work and enough education. School isn't the only way, but it is the surest way, especially for women, who are less equipped to advance through brute force. That is the equivalent of trying to succeed strictly by selling drugs, sports, rapping or pimping - brute force. The force of your determination, the force of your personality, and the force of your skills are with great limits without an education. Women have begun to use brute force more, theirs is her physicality. The belief that her nice body and pretty face is enough for her to get by is another form of brute force.

Blacks have increasingly high numbers in the rate of teenagers that drop out of high school. We have probably all heard that there are more Blackmen in jail than in college. These uneducated Blackmen will probably find low paying manual labor, work in construction or custodial, or try to hustle their way to prosperity. What options does a young lady uneducated and unskilled have? There are only so many video girls making a decent living beautifying the screen. It is no coincidence that we have had a rise in girls dropping out of school, and a rise in young ladies becoming strippers, prostitutes, and drug dealers. So women -stop shaking your ass, stop depending on the next American Gangster, stop thinking you are the next Halle Berry, Tyra Banks, or Buffy the Body because the guys around the way keep saying, " Damn You Fine ". Get an education so you can have some options in life. Get a formal education, because you need that to navigate this Capitalist System, but also get knowledge of self - knowledge of your real history and greatness, because you need that to navigate a world of whites trying to convince you that you are inferior to them.

We also have to educate our children, they will need computer skills, technological skills and entrepreneur skills to be able to build and maintain their own businesses. Knowledge is Power - that is knowledge of yourself, knowledge of the world around you, and knowledge of how to financially care for yourself and your loved ones. We need to get it in our children's head that for every 1 rich rapper that made it without a high school diploma, there is a thousand prisoners wishing they had one.

Unrealistic ideas and images our Black children have that education is no-longer needed is a reason why in the last 20 years, the number of Blackmen in prison has grown 500 percent. In 1980, there was 463,700 Blackmen in college and 143,000 Blackmen in prison. In 2,000 there were 603,032 in college and 791,600 Blackmen in prison. The numbers of lost, struggling, desperate and incarcerated Blackwomen are also outrageously high, because they are turning their backs on education, on knowledge, and on real Power.

Chapter 6

Assets vs. Possessions

Did you know that Blacks spend more money than any group in America? We don't make more, we don't have more, we don't save more, but we sure do spend more. While others make, hold, spend and save some. We have almost no hold mechanism - as soon as we get some money, we spend our money, and within hours our money is leaving our community and enriching the wallets and futures of other people.

In a study by John Wray, an economic development specialist in Washington, D.C, he traced the flow of dollars through comparative ethnic communities. The study showed that in the Asian community, a dollar circulates among the community's banks, brokers, shopkeepers, and business professionals for up to twenty-eight days before it is spent with outsiders. In the Jewish community, the circulation period was nineteen days. In the White Anglo-Saxon community, seventeen days was the circulation period. In the African-American community the circulation rate was a mere six hours/before our dollars were leaving our community to be in some other people's pocket.

Black people spend about 800 billion a year, and we are the greatest consumers of worthless possessions that go to waste, go out of style, and are over-priced trinkets and clothing to foster a richer than we are image. We spend all our money, damn near on nothing but possessions, while others are smart enough to spend their money on assets.

Possessions are items that don't increase in value, don't make you wealthier, takes money out your pocket and don't put shit in - like 20 pair of 200 dollar shoes, 3 cars, a drawer full of bull-shit jewelry, and every over-priced piece of new clothing a millionaire somewhere can slap a name brand on.

We need to make, hold, spend and save our money, too! We need to spend more of our money on assets and not just possessions. Interest earning account - asset, a wise purchase of property - asset, wise investments - asset, interest earning children's school fund - asset, classes and additional training leading to increase salary - asset, a small business - asset, rental property - asset. When we do spend our money, we need to shop wholesalers, discounters, close-outs, and direct distributors so we have more left over to purchase assets. We are spending the most on worthless bull-shit and paying the highest prices for it. Even our so-called celebrities and millionaires make a habit of having millions of dollars' worth of possessions and no real savings, investments, or substantial passive income. Passive income is something that makes you money even if you don't leave the bed that day - like royalties, real estate, and investments.

Power comes not from having many possessions, but from having plenty of assets. We need to stop spending our money enriching others. You never catch Jews or Asians spending their money with Blacks, and Whites try to avoid it as much as possible. Blacks spend enough money in America to be a wealthy Nation themselves, if we were smart enough to not send all our dollars to other people's bank account.

Blackwomen, you are the biggest consumers of goods in America. Madison Avenue advertisers know that if you make it, the Blacks will buy it - even if we don't advertise to them, they will find it anyway. We are so ridiculous with our money, we spend millions and billions of dollars with companies that more than disrespect us, they ridicule us in public and their ads. Companies like Timberland shoes and others will say, 'they don't want us in their clothes- it cheapens them' and we go ahead and spend more millions.

Even Jay-Z has recently campaigned against Cristal Champagne in his raps, saying they are racists. This is after him and the rap community increased Cristal's revenue by about 100 million dollars promoting their champagne for free, for years in their music and videos - mostly to poor Blacks who couldn't afford it. That's what we do; watch our celebrities promote the shit out of some other's people product, that don't even respect our communities. We go spend all our money on nonsense we can't afford, so they get rich and we stay poor. With the Web providing access to the whole world, there is no reason why we can't find goods and products made and owned by Black people all across the globe at a fraction of the prices these White people be charging us. At a fraction of the price and with better quality and creativity.

The number one goal has to be to stop giving our hard-earned money away to others, so they can take our money out of our communities and use it to enrich themselves, their community, their children, and their futures .

Besides keeping our money, we need to control our ability to earn money. One of the greatest assets is business ownership. Having your own business, even as a secondary source of income is very empowering. Entrepreneurship gives one the Power to control their earning ability and not be dependent on the whims of an employer. Business ownership has always been the most direct path to wealth and Power. Ownership also allows you to lobby politicians and contribute to the ones with interests and agendas that most benefit you and yours.

The hours you spend making others rich can be used to make you rich and being the sole-controller of your financial future is one of the greatest Powers. Plus, the big secret most people don't know is - if you structure a business   properly, you earn more, get more deductions get more benefits and pay much, less taxes.   For example if you were incorporated and earned up to 49,999 you would only pay 15 percent in Federal taxes.   If you were an individual that made 49,999 dollars, you would pay 25 percent in Federal taxes. That's why the rich get richer and the poor get poorer.

Another thing killing our pockets and our power to save money is these Pagan holidays with their savage histories that are used as a way to make store owners rich. Did you know that statistically, Black people are 99 percent consumers? Which means we produce less than 1 percent of the goods in this country. So in essence, our Black dollars keep the American economy prosperous - prosperous for them.

Now back to the savage holidays Black people insist on going in debt for every year. Let's start with the biggest trickery of your precious dollars - Christmas. The historical birth of Jesus Christ has no relationship to the date of December 25th.

The Nicaean Council at 325 A.D. met at the city of Nicaea (present day Turkey), on the mandate of Roman Emperor Constantine. They decided that the original Messiah Jesus ben Joseph, the Afro-Israelite (who was Black as night), would be Europeanized and his birth would be celebrated on December 25th to harmonize it with White people's most Pagan and popular holiday - Saturnalia. December 25th is supposed to be the birth of Saturn, a homosexual god. whitemen on that day would all get drunk, strip naked, have sex with each other and then go home and beat their wives. That's still how many whitemen practice Christmas and we Blacks are tricked into a year of debt, to get store owners rich and to celebrate a homosexual god.

Thanksgiving in America is the celebration of the Pilgrims who were saved from starvation by the Indians, and in return they slaughtered them - millions of them and that's what Americans are giving thanks for - mass extermination of Indians, and the mass enslavement and extermination of Blacks.

All holidays have origins not related to Black people and we refuse to save our money, and celebrate our own history in our own ways. Another example is Valentine's Day, which is the celebration of the execution of a priest in Ancient Rome named St. Valentine. St. Valentine was executed Feb. 14th, his heart cut out and placed in a box, because he defied the Emperor Claudius III orders. The Emperor decided to outlaw marriage for young men because he felt men without wives and families made better soldiers. St. Valentine continued marrying men to women and was executed for it. His death has now been made into an expensive holiday that put a lot of pressure on couples to buy expensive gift - to further enrich the pockets of another, not yourself or your lover.

So now that you know more about your so-called holidays, maybe you will find something more constructive to do with your money. At least spend your money on real assets (things that appreciate not depreciate) and stop wasting your money on mere possessions.

Chapter 7

Who You Are!

Ladies words have Power. When men, even your own men call you derogatory names, that's what they are trying to do - consciously" or unconsciously strip you of Power. You are not a hoe, never been a bitch, and are so much more than most want you to know. The word Bitch is so popular; it's almost a nick-name for Blackwomen in our music and culture. Bitch isn't a word we invented or should identify with. Bitch is a female dog and you know who worship the dog? The whiteman.

The savage whiteman while dwelling in caves in the early B.C. (Before Christ), fell in love with the dog and decided he would worship the dog. The savage whiteman was opposed to worshipping the only gods and goddesses of the only known religion at that time - The Blackman and Blackwoman and their religion. The whiteman named this animal dog out of disrespect, because its name is God spelled backwards. Even later, when 'the whiteman started its earliest civilization - Rome (1,000 B.C. villages, 250 B.C. town), it credited the founding of Rome to two brothers named Remus and Romulus, who were supposed to have been suckled and raised by wolves another kind of dog.

So now we use a word they invented to worship a filthy animal to denigrate our own women. We Blackmen have been so tricked; we can't even be original in our destructive ways - Sorry Blackwomen!

Remember, the very first Goddess worshipped was You - The Blackwoman (Isis). The very first Madonna and Child was You (Isis and Horus). The very first Queens, inventors, civilizers, and teachers were you. The Blackwoman was and is The Mother of Civilization and there's no-one greater. You have always been worth more than your hips and thighs, your ass and grind. Through the ages men have tried to hold you down, hold you back, box you in, but no box can hold you. It's time you knew the real you and continue to be that again.

Despite their most persistent and egregious efforts, they cannot hide the fact that You - The Blackwoman is The Mother of Civilization. Every religion and culture was built with your intelligence and righteousness as their foundation. Greatness, spiritual beauty and divine wisdom run all through your veins. Every one of you is to be respected and held in very high esteem, but it starts with you. Blackwomen have to demand respect with their ways and actions and in what treatment they will accept from others.

Be all that you are - Beautiful, Powerful, Wise, and Righteous. That Is your history, your legacy and your true identity.

Science reports that everyone alive today descended
from an Afrikan woman who lived 200,000 years ago!

Based on the evidence of recent findings, modern (white) science has
'officially' declared that ALL of present humanity came from one race...the
Black race –the oldest race. Throughout the world prominent magazines have
done front page articles on "the most incredible find of all times: Scientists
have unearthed the ancient bones of a Black African [Pygmy] woman who is

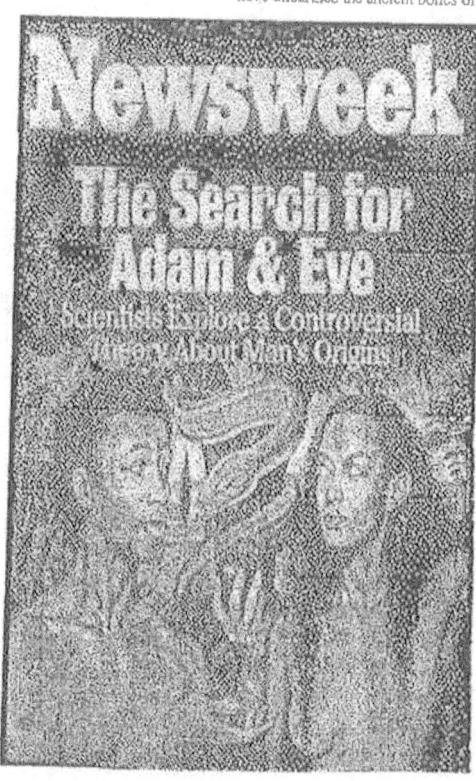

indisputably the mother of all
humanity!"

They nicknamed her *Eve*, "our
common ancestor –a woman who
–lived 200,000 years ago and left
resilient genes that are carried by all of
mankind" reports the bestselling issue
ever of *Newsweek* magazine (1/11/88),
which depicts a Black Adam and Eve
on its front cover, headlining it *The
Search for Adam and Eve*.

Science magazine (9/11/87) stated that
overwhelming evidence shows that
"Africa was the cradle of modern
humans... The story the molecular
biology seems to be telling is that
modern humans evolved in Africa
about 200,000 years ago."

National Geographic (Oct. 88) reports
of new evidence "of an African origin
for modern humans."

Not only did You - the mighty and magnificent Women of Color give
birth to all of humanity, you participated in the birth of all the
sciences that are still used today.

New Debate Over Humankind's Ancestress

Biologists insist all human lineages track back to a woman in Africa 200,000 years ago.

By NATALIE ANGIER

HE may no longer be called Eve, and her most imaginative and outspoken proponent may have died two months ago, but the provocative notion that our genes hold evidence of a mother of us all is growing ever more powerful.

By this theory on the origins of modern Homo sapiens, all 5.384 billion humans on Earth today can be traced to a woman who lived in Africa about 200,000 years ago, and who left an unmistakable if wraithlike signature on our DNA.

The woman was a member of a race of the first truly modern people, who, with their newly lightened skeletons, their more capacious brains and their softer brows, radiated out from their African homeland and overwhelmed or supplanted the many more primitive humans who were then living in Asia and Europe.

Tracing Descent Back to a Genetic Eve

Tree based on analysis of genetic sequences in 189 people of diverse races; it shows a common female ancestor in Africa, 166,000 to 249,000 years ago.

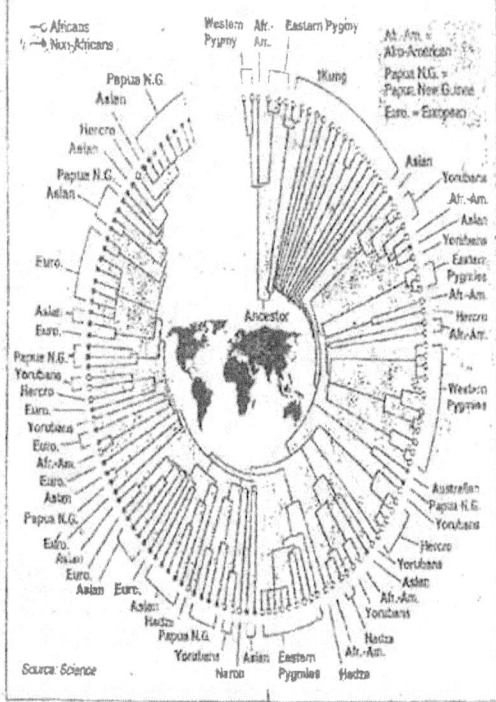

Source: Science

The New York Times

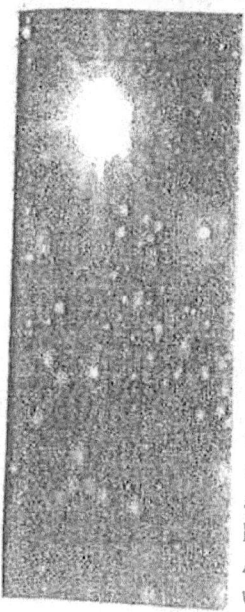

The ancient Afrikans (mainly Black women) originated and developed what I call "StarScience," for the artificial separation we know as Astrology and Astronomy did not exist until the Europeans got a hold of it. Climatically, geographically, and agriculturally, Afrika was the ideal location on Earth for the birth of StarScience. StarScience itself is evidence of the vast antiquity of Afrika civilization. StarScience must be at least 52,000 years old (length of 2 Precessions), since it was mapped out by direct observation. The Zodiac could only be charted in the sky after the Great Year (Precession or revolution of the Zodiac) had been determined. StarScience is the Mother of Sciences, probably millions of years old, for advanced Afrikan civilization stretches back millions of years. Simplicius (6th cent. A.D.) wrote that the Egyptians had kept astronomical observations and records for the last 630,000 years. The Kamite priests and priestesses distributed their zodiacal science, along with their life-honoring matriarchal culture around the world. Later volumes of this book address StarScience as the foundation of world civilization, agriculture, religion, mathematics, geometry, computer science. Only recently have Europeans partly caught up with the advanced knowledge which the Afrikan Dogon people possess concerning StarScience and awareness of stars which are only visible through the most technically advanced telescopes.

The origin of all religions started in Africa with the Blackman and Black-woman. Egyptian Religion and mythology-is the source of all deities, stories, themes, rituals, prayers, symbols, and teachings of the world's religions. Christianity, Islam, and Judaism all have their foundation in Egypt. All the stories of the Bible originated from the allegories of Egypt (Kamit), which are stories of the Twa People (called Pygmies by Europeans). Over a hundred thousand years before Christianity, the Twa People taught about heaven, about a Christ born of a virgin and dying for their sins. Every culture and people imitated the gods and goddesses of Egypt; especially the Madonna and Child.

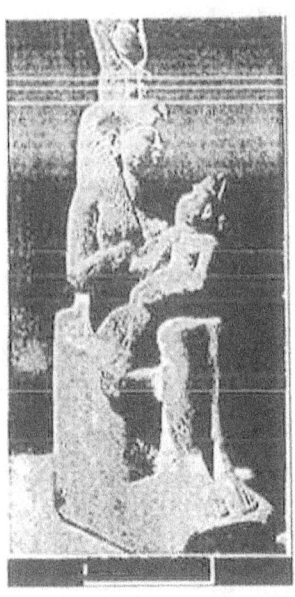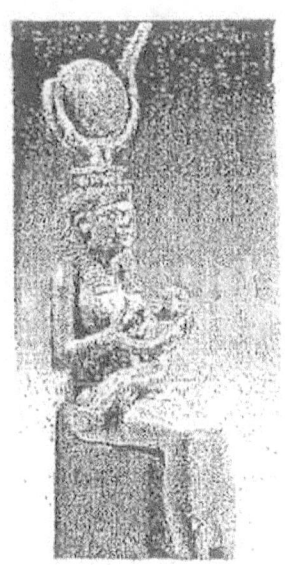

Actually the worship of the virgin, Black "Mother of God" with her God-begotten child, far predates Christianity and prevailed throughout the ancient world.

Historians recognize that the statue of the Egyptian Goddess Isis with her child Horus in her arms was the first Madonna and Child. They were renamed Mary and Jesus when Europe was forcibly Christianized. The worship of Isis and Horus was especially popular in ancient Rome. "Roman legions carried this figure of Black Isis holding the Black infant Horus all over Europe where shrines were established to her. So holy and venerate were these shrines that when Christianity invaded Europe, these figures of the Black Isis holding the Black Horus were not destroyed but turned into figures of the Black Madonna and Child. Today these are still the holiest shrines in Catholic Europe.'" Titles such as Our Lady, The Great Mother, are the same titles attributed to Isis. The word "Madonna" itself is from mater domina, a title used for Isis! The month of May, which was dedicated to the heathen Virgin Mothers, is also the month of Mary, the Christian Virgin.

Long before the Blackwoman was demonstrating her magnificence by being tennis greats like Venus and Serena. Before being dynamic television hosts and owners like Oprah and Debra Lee. Before being relentless freedom fighters like Harriet Tubman and Sojourner Truth. Before our Blackwomen were showing unbelievable strength and perseverance by surviving over 400 years of slavery while steadily holding our families together, and continuing to be incredible mothers, teachers, wives and societal builders - The Blackwoman was Queens and warriors.

Like Queen Hatshepsut who reigned over Egypt and many other lands from 1515 to 1484 B.C.E.

The Only Queen In History Officially Listed As A King

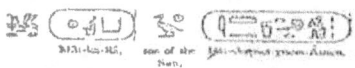

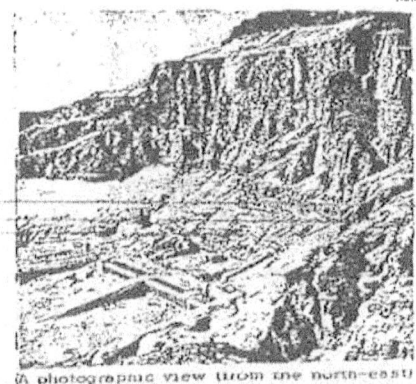

A photographic view (from the north-east) of the ruins of Queen Hatshepsut's Funerary at Luxor (Thebes) or Deir el-Bahri.

The splendor of Egypt's architecture is best exhibited in this structure. Modern public buildings fall short of its beauty and colossal magnitude.

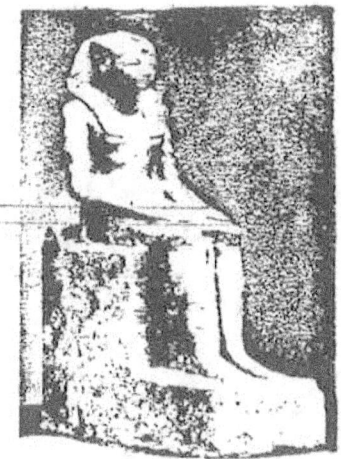

HAT-SHEP-SUT, XVIIIth Dynasty, c. 1515 - 1484, the FIRST QUEEN in history to rule over a nation. Limestone statue, Museum of Art.

QUEEN HATSHEPSUT'S EXPEDITION TO THE LAND OF PUNT.

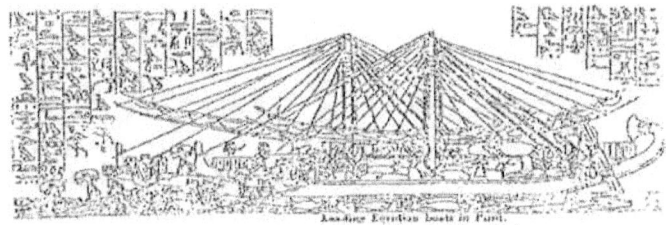

Other powerful female Queens ruled lands and were at the height of politics, before we had the awesome examples of Ellen Johnson-Shirleaf, present President of Liberia;-and our very own Michelle Obama - First Lady extraordinaire.

Like Queen (Empress) Makeda, affectionately known as Queen of Sheba, who ruled over Ethiopia (Kush), for many, many years. She protected her lands, treated her people justly, held back foreign invaders and even have her meeting with King Solomon reported in the Bible; 1 Kings 10:1-13.

There were also fearless rulers like Queen Nzinga of Angola, who fought against the Portuguese slave traders between 1630 and 1648.

Then we have one of our most famous ancient Queens; Nefertiti. She was wife of Akhenaton, she helped rule Egypt and she was unmistakably African woman.

Even Europe was taught royalty by the Blackwoman.
Europe's royal families descended from Black / Mulatto rulers!
This makes sense when you know that Afrikans ruled in Europe for 1400 years. Afrikans introduced the concept of royalty to the Europeans, who were initially uncivilized barbarians. Afrikan ancestry in Europeans is well documented in Nature Knows No Color Line, by J.A. Rogers. To list a few:

1. the Black Queen Charlotte Sophia, the grandmother of Queen Victoria, who was also the consort and the great-great-grandmother of George VI.
2. Jean Baptiste Bernadotte who founded the present day royal Swedish family
3. The Duke of Florence
4. The Medicis, the Gonzagas
5. The Duchess of Alafoes
6. St. Hilaire-son of Louis XV

...long is the list! Is this why some of Europe's oldest royal/ noble families are called the "Black Nobility" even though they're "white"?

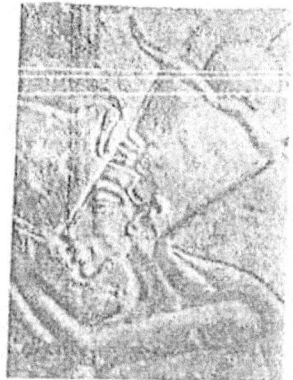

Despite images of this great Queen looking Europeanized, she was an African Woman. This is a true depiction of her, as found on ancient Egyptian temple walls. She was a true Blackwoman, running shit, even her Husband/King; young Akhenaton.

Carvings Give Nefertiti Big Role

By DONALD JANSON

Special to The New York Times

PHILADELPHIA, Jan. 8 — History has short-changed Queen Nefertiti of ancient Egypt's Golden Age by stressing only her beauty, Ray Winfeld Smith, an archeologist, believes.

The young queen may well have wielded the major religious, political and economic power of the day, he said in an interview.

If so, he namely Nefertiti was influential in establishing what was probably the world's first single-god religion, the worship of the sun disk Aten.

She may also have guided a change to greater naturalism in Egyptian art.

Both developments of the mid-14th century B.C. have been attributed to her husband, the summery King Akhenaten (or Ikhnaton). But Mr. Smith said his studies in Egypt for the last five years point to a far bigger role for Nefertiti than ever before accorded her.

She may not only have been the brains in the family, he said, but may also have done without the aid of him in conceiving their six daughters.

Carvings Analyzed

Mr. Smith based his observations on his analysis of carvings of about 35,000 stones of a temple to Aten that the youthful pharaoh had built at Karnak in the Egyptian capital of Thebes early in his 17-year reign.

The archeologist, a research associate at the University of Pennsylvania, here, headed a team that has used photographs and computers to reconstruct the pictures carved on the temple's scattered sandstone wall blocks so be seen and studied in proper relationship to each other rather than in fragments. Sponsors of the project include the museum, the Smithsonian Institution, and the Department of Antiquities of the United Arab Republic.

The temple was razed by a successor of Akhenaton after it stood for only two decades. The Smith team found individual blocks in museums and in private hands throughout Europe and in the United States. Many others had been pilfered by excavators in warehouses in Karnak or in the open at fill in monuments built in Karnak or in the open.

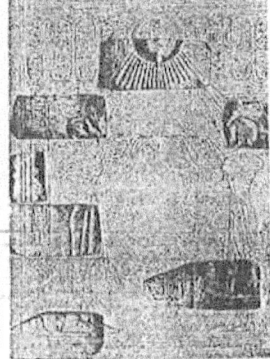

Reconstruction of wall at Karnak Temple, using the few available sandstone blocks, shows two figures—both Nefertiti—making an offering to Aten, sun disk god.

Queen Nefertiti

Luxor. Since the demolition of the temple, many of these had been used as foundations and fill in monuments built in her femininity.

Thebes by rulers who did not share Akhenaten's monotheistic view of religion.

Massive Jigsaw Puzzle

Mr. Smith, just back from Egypt to publish a book on his findings, said the 35,000 pieces of the massive jigsaw puzzle has been put together amounted to only 15 per cent of the original structure but enough to establish Nefertiti's preeminence to her day.

Images of the queen rather than the king dominated the temple carvings. An entire courtyard was devoted exclusively to her. Never before had a temple in the country's capital so emphasized a woman over the king, Mr. Smith said.

A century earlier a queen had ruled Egypt, but she disguised herself by wearing a beard. Nefertiti, whose name means "the beauty has come" retained in her femininity.

Each Egyptian king was god-like as well as secular ruler, but the temple drawings showed that Nefertiti assumed her husband's religious stature. She was revered as a goddess.

Depictions of the holiest of ritualistic ceremonies of the time, the offering of a treasured object to Aten, show twice as many god statues of Nefertiti used in the ceremonies as statues of her husband.

Egyptian additional prayers to Nefertiti. No other queen, Mr. Smith said, was accorded divinity while her husband lived. The richness of her role, he said, was not known before the pieces of the temple puzzle were put together.

Additional Evidence

Mr. Smith said supplementary evidence of Nefertiti's standing can be found at Tel-el Amarna, 240 miles down the Nile from Thebes, where Akhenaten built a new capital and dedicated it to Aten. An inscription on a stone boundary pillar reports that the queen had an idea of her own about building the city. Never before in Egyptian history, the archeologist said, had there been a recorded confession that a queen ever revealed ideas different from those of her husband.

Mr. Smith said he interprets some of the evidence to say that the tributes to Nefertiti at Karnak were not the result of the initiative of an adoring husband but flowed from her own sharpness personality.

He noted that existing literature gives the revolutionary ideas giving credit for the religious and cultural innovations of the day and for a powerful personality and intellect to her but this was done without proof.

He pointed out that portraits and busts of Akhenaten from the temple showed him as a king himself has thick, slender thighs and middle legs, apparently the result of a glandular disease.

Syndrome Cited

Persons born with such a syndrome, he said, are not likely to be particularly intelligent and tend to be early in disposition. He believes Nefertiti held strong sway over him and her subjects from the time they married at teen-agers till the young Pharaoh died in his 30's after a reign of 17 years.

This is only a fraction of the greatness Women of Color have surging through' their veins. This is only a small glimpse of the astounding accomplishments made manifest by you - the Original Women. To be phenomenal is your birthright, to be amongst you -is our privilege. So hold your head high and know that the essence of you has always been, is today, and will always be - Beautiful, Powerful, Wise and Righteous.

CHAPTER 8

The Sterilization of Puerto Rico

One of the most insidious methods of robbing Women of Color, of their power to build for the future has been sterilization. Through-out history and continued today, oppressive and racist systems have tried to deny poor women and Women of Color the choice and ability to have children. In Africa, Brazil, China, India, and all across Latin America, governments have participated in Eugenics programs designed to limit or remove a woman's ability to have children. The United States have initiated, supported and encouraged many sterilization over the years, but none as sinisterly successful as the sterilization programs in Puerto Rico. One-third of the Puerto Rican women of child-bearing age was sterilized by a U.S. sponsored system that deemed them unfit and their offspring undesirable, because they were Women of Color.

For over a hundred years America has used forced, illegal, deceptive, and discriminatory tactics to sterilize people Whites have judged as unwanted, unfit, undesirable and non-beneficial to them. In the 1870s Malthusianists and White nativist Protestants created a Eugenics program that led to the adoption of national and state policy. Between 1907 - 45 over 45,000 Americans considered mentally challenged were forcibly sterilized. In most major cities, including New York, it has been an unwritten policy to perform elective hysterectomies on poor Black and Puerto Rican women. Black and Puerto Rican women were and are pressured by the medical community to have hysterectomies; not to cure their supposed illness, but to control their child-bearing.

Other ways America forces sterilization is by threatening Women of Color with the loss of welfare benefits if they don't submit to various forms of Eugenics. When hysterectomies can't be coerced, the U.S. accomplish the same goal with mandating or encouraging the use of drugs to stop child-birth; like Norplant, Depo-Provera, or contraceptive vaccines like quinacrine. Similar sterilization campaigns resulted in the sterilization of 25 percent of Indian Women living on reservations in the 1970s.

Even though I advocate smart family planning when possible to increase a woman's and her child's chances at the very best quality of life; I don't think anyone has the right to deny a woman her chance at motherhood. The U.S. has sponsored and initiated some of the most devious, deceptive and destructive sterilization programs in history. Almost every sterilization program has targeted Women of Color, here in the United States and any territory the U.S. has great influence over. Even the United States second wealthiest man, Warren Buffet said on television that a large portion of his wealth was being donated to organizations for population control. Too many times, population control has meant the destruction and denial of Women of Color, the ability to bear children. Under the guise of population control, one third of Puerto Rican women were forced, pressured, coerced, financially influenced or deceived into being sterilized.

In the 1930s Puerto Rico was 80 percent Catholic and providing birth-control services was illegal. Soon afterwards campaigns were started to convince the people of Puerto Rico and specifically poor families that over-population was the blame for economic troubles, unemployment, and poverty. At the times over-population was being blamed for poverty, the real reason was - less than 2% of the population owned 80% of the land.

In 1937, a bill was signed that no-longer made birth-control services illegal, and 23 clinics were open to provide services to prevent pregnancy. Another bill was passed that authorized the Commission of Health in Puerto Rico to regulate the teachings and dissemination of eugenics principles and contraceptives to hospitals and health centers; this was followed by the opening of 160 more birth-control clinics. Then the U.S. passed law #136 that legalized sterilization for reasons other than strict medical need, and sterilization started being provided and encouraged to Puerto Rican women by physicians as the favored means of birth-control.

In 1939 the U.S. government started sending enormous amounts of money to P.R. for birth-control programs and encouraged women to accept sterilization by providing it at minimal cost or free. At the same time, U.S. manufacturing companies needed cheap labor on the Island, and women were coerced into getting sterilized, so they would be free of childcare and able to get employment. To the U.S., Puerto Rico was an excellent source of cheap labor, high profits tax-free business opportunities and a testing ground for their population control programs. The media promoted a over-population hysteria, propaganda film clips were shown in the U.S. in the 1940s, 50s, 60s and 70s to further convince people over-population was the culprit of all Puerto Rico's problem and that sterilization was the cure.

Of the three areas, political, legal and medical - it was the medical community that did the most damage. In Puerto Rico physicians are highly revered, almost like saints and their word rarely challenged. The physicians started pushing sterilization as birth-control, because many felt Puerto Rican women were too dumb to understand other contraceptive methods. Most women weren't told of other contraceptive options, weren't told that it required surgery, and weren't told the operation was irreversible. Another common practice was to persuade any woman following child-birth, while medicated, in pain and exhausted to agree to sterilization. In one small town, Barceloneta, 20,000 women were sterilized between 1956 and 1976. There were no restrictions on age, health or whether they had children already and few women were fully informed of the surgery and its effect. In Puerto Rico, "La Operacion" was the term used to identify this widely available and popular means of birth-control.

Not only was P.R. a testing ground for population control thru sterilization, but also a testing laboratory for birth-control pills as well. In 1956, the first birth-control pills were tested on Puerto Rican women living in government housing, these pills were 20 times stronger than the pills eventually used in the U.S. 30 years later. Many women became ill, yet doctors and nurses continued giving them to women, sometimes even going door to door persuading women to take them as part of a family planning program. These women were unaware they were being used as guinea pigs by the medical community and pharmaceutical companies, with the blessings of the United States government.

By 1980, Puerto Rico had the highest rate of female sterilization in the whole world. Munoz Marin, founder of the Popular Democratic Party and former governor in Puerto Rico announced his support for family planning programs (sterilization), he said, "even if it must be carried out with the necessary muscle". Sterilization, backed by the U.S., was indeed targeted to the poor and uneducated and was never a truly 'voluntary' choice, because it was never a truly 'informed' choice. Even public schools in P.R. drilled it in the heads of children, that having small families practically guaranteed financial stability and a more prosperous life - like the White, happy American families pictured in their school books.

Despite the aggressive sterilization programs implemented through-out Puerto Rico, inflation rose and unemployment skyrocketed. In the 70's, half of the population in P.R. was on food stamps, 60% of the people lived below the poverty line, and the profits of U.S. companies in P.R. had grown by 500%. The U.S. was and still remains impervious to the rights, health and economic status of poor people and especially Women of Color. The U.S. main objective is profits and power and the oppression and exploitation of Puerto Rican people is just one more example of that. The Eugenics program initiated and supported by U.S. policy has been one of the most insidious, blatantly racist programs ever, resulting in the sterilization of a record one-third of the female population at one time. Once again, Women of Color are being robbed of their power; their power to build, their power to decide, their power to be -be their very best, be their most powerful, and be able to define themselves - for themselves.

Chapter 9

Latinas, Abused and Ignored

In countries around the world women suffer atrocious abuse at the hands of their lovers, mates, and husbands. Women in Mexico and Central America suffer abuse from their mates and indifference from their governments. Many of these women seek asylum to escape the dangers and is confronted by another kind of indifference. Like the documented case of a woman who was beaten and raped by her husband for over 20 years and even when she tried to leave him - gunmen were sent to shoot-up her home. When she was pregnant he attempted to kill her by choking her and when he had tired of his four daughters, he even tried to drown them. Despite such threats of death, this Guatemalan woman could get no help from police after several visits and the various government offices she complained to refused to help her. It is the case for many women in Mexico and Central America that when they are being abused, raped or threatened with death by their mates that no-one listens to them. Those women brave enough and lucky enough to escape the constant violence at home to seek asylum in the United States often face the same kind of indifference they tried to escape. Under current laws, most women like the Guatemalan woman fleeing for her life and the lives of her four daughters, they will lose their U.S. asylum case and be sent back home.

Last year, about 40,000 people from all over the world applied for asylum in the United States. Only one in four people seeking asylum in the U.S. are granted protection. For Latinos and especially Latina women, the numbers are far less. On average, more than 3,000 Guatemalans apply for asylum and 95 percent are turned away and forced to return to their country. For Salvadorans, 97 percent are denied asylum and sent back home, and for Mexicans 98 percent are denied asylum and sent back to their violence infested countries.

In Mexico and Central America, the violence has reached epidemic proportions. The whole region is experiencing bloodshed at a level far greater than any part of the world not in a war zone. For the women of this region, the dangers are even worse. Case, after case, after case shows that women in Mexico and Central America can be abused, raped, even killed with an almost accepted impunity. In these various countries, the deadly combination of machismo, police corruption and government inefficiency is a breeding ground for the continued violence and abuse against women that goes virtually unpunished.

In documented cases Mexican and Central American women have testified they were refused any assistance from police, government officials, even judges; unless they gave them sex first. In Guatemala, United Nations and private foundation research shows that at least one in three women suffers domestic violence, while hundreds are murdered by their partners every year. In Guatemala and many Latin countries, police and court protection is a rarity. Of 10,000 cases, only 1,000 will be reported, only 10 will be investigated, and maybe one will result in conviction; according to Amanda Martin, director of the Guatemalan Human Rights Commission, a non-profit organization in Washington, D.C.

Despite growing mounds of evidence proving the severe abuse women suffer, asylum in the U.S. still remains a hurdle very few Latina women could overcome. Even a woman that could prove she had been pistol-whipped and beaten unconscious by her husband, only secured asylum after a fifteen year legal battle. Meeting the legal definition needed to obtain asylum in the U.S. is these endangered women's' biggest challenge.

To gain asylum, immigrants must be facing grave dangers in their own country, a threat that an internal relocation won't eliminate. They must also prove that their government has either harmed them or refused to protect them. Then the third requirement is showing they are in danger because of their race, religion, nationality, political opinion or membership in a particular social group.
Even with The Obama Administration making abused women eligible for asylum, which reversed the Bush Administration's earlier stance against allowing abused women asylum; escape from abuse, violence, rape and even murder, still remain a dream most Latina women never obtain.

There are recent cases that give some hope. A recent California ruling in the case of Lesly Yajayra Perdomo, did say that Guatemalan women should be considered a social group. Also, in august 2010, a Mexican woman won asylum after showing that Mexican officials failed to protect her from severe, long-term abuse inflicted by her husband. However, these cases are not precedent and not binding, so other officials could still decide in other ways and continue to deny most abused women the much needed protection they seek.

These Latina women represent another group of women of Color being abused and neglected, not only by their men, their own country, but also a U.S. court system ran by a bunch of insensitive, weak-moraled men. Until we learn to stand-up for mothers, wives, daughters and Women of Color everywhere - our own women will remain vulnerable to the abuses perpetrated on women of Color everywhere, everyday!

The History of Abuses and The Need for Asylum have always been detrimental to the lives of People of Color, especially Women of Color. When proper love and relationships can be found, a powerful tool in the survival and success of Women of Color.

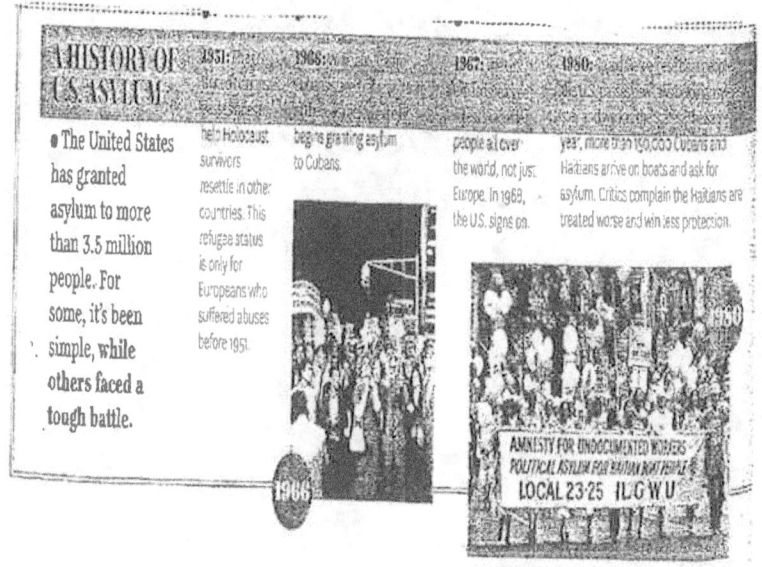

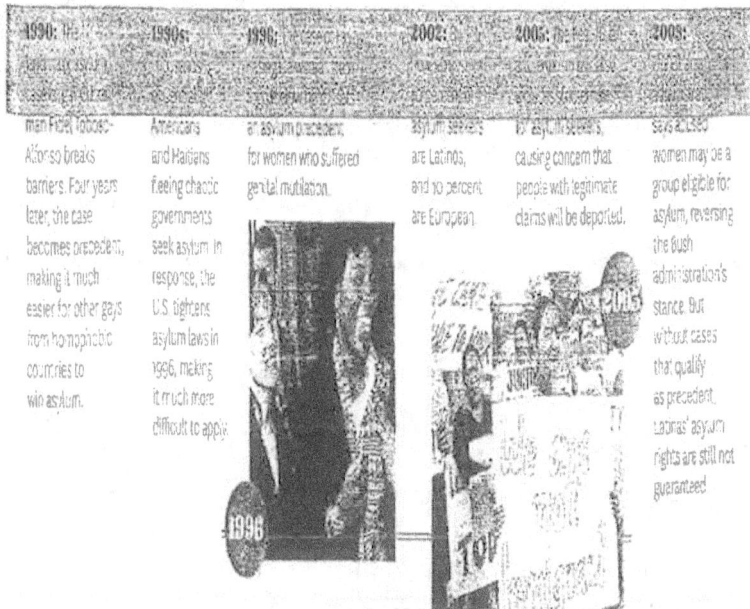

| 1990: ... | 1990s: ... | 1996: ... | 2002: ... | 2005: ... | 2009: ... |

man Fidel Toboso-Alfonso breaks barriers. Four years later, the case becomes precedent, making it much easier for other gays from homophobic countries to win asylum.

Americans and Haitians fleeing chaotic governments seek asylum. In response, the U.S. tightens asylum laws in 1996, making it much more difficult to apply.

an asylum precedent for women who suffered genital mutilation.

asylum seekers are Latinos, and 10 percent are European.

to asylum seekers, causing concern that people with legitimate claims will be deported.

says abused women may be a group eligible for asylum, reversing the Bush administration's stance. But without cases that qualify as precedent, Latinas' asylum rights are still not guaranteed.

1996

PART TWO

I kiss the earth, I am the sun.
She needs my warmth radiating sure and steady,
She reaches for me; glistens and clothes herself in
sincerity to honor my presence.

I kiss the earth, I am the cloud
She becomes quiet and receptive to the soft drops of rain
that I whisper to her.
And to the downpour that could reach and alter her core.
She yields to flood waters that remove obstacles, creating
paths to fruitful new mornings.

In a dry season she misses water, even for tears. In a
deluge she begs my strength to bear the burden
And I answer with a kiss familiar and true.
I am the heaven she moves in,
Whenever I shine my light on you.

Introduction

To Powerful Relationships

We are into a new decade and we face some unique challenges - some delightful and some depressing. Despite a recession, Women of Color, especially Blacks,   have never been so influential and so affluent in America. It's hard for anyone to deny that You have become the standard of beauty, strength, and innovation in America. With or without a partner you lead - our culture, our communities, and our homes.

I want to see all our women flourish even more. I want to see you powerful, within yourself and within our Nation. I want to see you women successfully guide our children through the obstacles, to propagate an even greater future of great accomplishments. I truly want to see you very deserving women happy and full of love - receiving and giving love in the most fruitful and productive ways.

To be your best, all you have to do is reach deep inside of you and grab the priceless jewels buried inside of you since forever. You are a sparkling example of feminine divineness and before I end this conversation, I want to help you find someone to appreciate it.

You are and will continue to be phenomenal in all your endeavors, with or without a mate. Power can be obtained alone, but it's so much harder, and to be powerfully happy - Women of Color / Mother of Civilization / Queen Earth, usually wants a good man by her side.

On this subject of Powerful Relationships, I thought it would benefit you to have a few different perspectives. I enlisted the help of three diverse, strong, and intelligent Blackwomen to offer their views on finding the right man and developing a Powerful Relationship.

It is my sincere hope and belief that their shared love and triumphs, failures, experiences and expectations can help you in your Quest. I have shared my knowledge, now share in their wisdom.

WISDOM
PROLOGUE

With as much honesty and humility resulting from personal experience, hard-earned lessons, and heart-felt responsibility to our community as a black woman, I answer my brother's appeal to look and light a way for finding black love. With the idealism of a new love, the fluency and familiarity of old friends, the depth and reality of our past, present and possibly our future, you the reader, are being asked to truly consider the ideas that have already been posited and those that will be discussed now from a woman's perspective.

For many women this dialogue isn't new, it has occurred many times under conditions as varied as the emotions—anger, infatuation, guilt, betrayal, desire, regret, fear, disillusionment—that usually infuse it. In most of these common exchanges we share and walk away consciously intent on stringing together however many pearls of wisdom the last love experience provided us, hoping that their value is real and will be appreciated for us and be appreciated by the next man that we decide to love. Other times we come to the end of an experience completely oblivious to any value gained. Acutely aware instead, of only the losses that were sustained. Confusing that awareness and disillusionment with truth—the truth of who we are and what we should learn to expect in return when we present our hearts. We end up going forward inadvertently tainting future prospects for others and ourselves. The disillusionment may, but the truth is not supposed to hurt.

What can be new in this instance is that the authentic truth concerning how we engage in love can be acknowledged as the clarion-call that it is meant to be and allowed to heal previously held misconceptions. It can be a call to make real adjustments to the standpoint from which we approach or even just consider one another in the interest of love. For the health and continued existence of our race and culture this instance can be a salve that enables us to see the need and learn to recognize the connection between the seemingly inconsequential, strictly personal choices that we make and actions that we take in our lives and the far-reaching impact that those things have had and will have on our collective experience. As already suggested in the first half of this book, before we're able to make any worthy connection beyond our individual selves we have to truly connect with our individual selves as women not girls, not even as ladies and certainly not any of the nonsense personas that are constantly offered up for our choosing. Women have to present in our relationships if we expect men to show forth.

"To be treated like a Queen you gotta reach a certain point too, at that destination a King will anoint you." Common

—Carol Blades

CHAPTER 10

The Lovin' at Sunrise

Our love relationships, seven years into this new millennia, suffer more blight than many of us can stand to acknowledge. While some within our community have managed to stay head above the troubled waters of our frayed bonds by making up their minds to commit to solid, nurturing marriages, or long secure unions, the distractions from healthy unions are many, very attractive and often welcomed alternatives.

Probing beyond the 'no good men' war cry that women dare men to challenge or deny, we need to determine what standards we've been employing. This is necessary to determine not only what a good man should be, but just as importantly, what standards have we set for ourselves to be recognized as good women. The time is ripe for us to look honestly at ourselves in order to play our part in bringing about positive changes in the way that we love. Our tendency to trivialize or oversimplify the causes and reality of being single, have many of us 'starving in the midst of plenty'.

There are numerous things that weigh into so many Black women being single. Namely, the attitudes that we espouse, the choices that we make repeatedly, and the circumstances that we contend with as a result, can be counted among the ways that we contribute, by default, to the hardships that single women experience. Whether it's the case that we are single and wanting, single and satisfied or single and scared as hell, without asking critical questions of ourselves, the emotional and familial isolation that exists in the Black community will remain unreasonably pervasive and commonplace, transcending our individual realities and casting shadows on our future progress as a whole.

One of the most basic detriments to our solidarity that needs to be confronted is the tendency that we have of being a hindrance to one another due to carelessness in how we interact. It should be noted here that there are undoubtedly women who while single by choice, remain optimistic to the possibility of at some point sharing a love and commitment with an especially exquisite man. These women have more than likely discarded the poison-laced delusion of how that love would come to be for a more fulfilling ideal based on the practicality of taking care of home first. Many times we fail to approach relationships with the level of sobriety that would better enable us to empower ourselves and our people by building on our strengths instead of settling for low expectations. Despite living in one of the most affluent countries in the world at a most advantageous time, many in our community continue to struggle in very real ways that eclipse the ability to benefit from America's wealth of opportunity in ways beyond day to day survival. Instead our pursuits are reduced to very individualistic efforts as we find ourselves having just enough to think and act only on behalf of our-selves or our immediate family and friends. In the most desperate situations this reaction is forced upon us as a result of limited resources—financial, educational, or medical. The inability to cope or effectively withstand the persistence of these influences makes it hard to grasp broader possibilities and imposes a heavy emotional and mental toll on an individual. Lost are the opportunities to develop and make full use of our talents and abilities and become effectual models in our community.

For women in particular who are often not only the sole providers for dependent children, but also for ailing parents or other relatives we look to the men in our lives, sometimes after the fact, to help us in bearing the weight of these types of situations. Often it's only to find that through their misguided actions coupled with our own, they've in the end only added to the distress and instability of the situation. Very easily we find ourselves dealing with effects of the blind leading the blind because no precise assessment of what is available or what is lacking has been determined individually and agreed upon mutually by the couple. This point is an important one because initially women desire to be good and right and supportive of our men. When we believe that their intentions toward us are the same, working together makes perfect sense on the face of things. If however what is needed or desired isn't clearly conveyed from the beginning, it's really easy for the reasons and the ways that we are together as couples to become blurred. And absence of communication is the easiest way to set ourselves up to fall short of overcoming the initial difficulties that can be expected when problems arise, that they were lied to or taken advantage of when in reality there can't honestly be any claims of deception, abuse or blame to be exacted if no goals or guidelines were established in the first place. And because there seems to be some inherent reluctance among Black men and women to speak plainly to each other, this is typically the point at which the faultfinding begins. This is when everything that we wanted to say but only expressed to our girlfriends instead of him, everything that we felt uneasy about but went ahead and did anyway comes to the fore. We start to see our man, our husband, our child's father, our counterpart, our love—as the embodiment of everything that has ever made our hearts ache, part and parcel of everything that has ever challenged us to show proof of our worth and value as a Black female since we were young. We feel fearful that we are in fact alone in all the good that we desire and are willing to sacrifice for on behalf of our men, our children and ourselves.

Of course there are those of us that have been spared the first-hand knowledge of wanting for anything materially, but still possess the selfish mindset that is easily associated with sustained hardship. Only in this instance the hardship may be more emotional in nature. Even in these situations there are women trying very simply to add the enjoyment of companionship to their otherwise stable lifestyle but instead find men that are all too willing to take advantage of their situation no matter how finely balanced it is on the precipice of gainful employment, or family privilege. But these are also likely to be the times in which equipped with moderately better means and options we ourselves become the perpetrators of the fractured relationships among Black men and women.

There are women that expend considerable time and energy hating, hurting and trying to hinder men in any way that they can, as if this were a plausible way to be validated as a woman. When we women are the ones doing wrong it is often, as it is in the case with men, at the suggestion and encouragement of our friends. For instance it may seem a benign indulgence to do things like having unprotected sex once or twice with someone while we are or have the knowledge that they are seriously involved with someone else. Or act in similar fashion with someone who isn't involved with anyone because of all the craziness that he has going on all by himself. Less benign are the more celebrated instances of scheming on some dude's money. Rarely is the situation in these cases as desperate as it's made to seem in effort to justify the actions. Why is it never apparent in all of the giddy excitement of our master plan how low we'll feel on the other side of 'money-in-hand!? When the money is gone but he's still agonizing over why the alleged abortion was even necessary. Or when the room is paid for but the pillow talk centers on old girl and how she is catching feelings. There is of course any number of scenarios that easily lead one way or another to hurt feelings, compromised self-esteem, actual unplanned pregnancies and other more profound outcomes that we find ourselves dealing with longer than intended. Some women are in no way subtle or indirect in their conniving conduct and could give a damn about an outcome. The women that do care and will most likely be present to feel it when the consequences game out, still remain to some degree resistant to accepting any culpability in the situations or how they contribute to why so many of us ultimately find ourselves alone as single women or single mothers.

While having already acknowledged the existence of tri-fling men among us, the learned adversarial manner and animosity that both genders perpetuate in the Black community has to cease. Beyond the anemic love between Black men and women we have to start being more supportive in our friendships as well. We women have to stop encouraging each other in small-minded behavior. Stop jealously, viciously attempting to erode the efforts of our friends in trying to establish and maintain healthy relationships. This will require that we offer our comments less often, more conscientiously and without tainting the advice with our own embittered experiences. For those that are in relationships, learn to share the business more selectively, if at all. Without undercutting the incomparable value of sister friends among Black women, we have to learn to temper our belief that everyone that we've found reason to call a friend has your best interest at heart. As grown women we should at the very least be able to state what's on our minds to the man we claim to be with without having to first get a consensus from our girls. Even in the event that the relationship with him ends or is by all other accounts shot to hell, try to avoid telling it all especially if it's something you can work out yourself. Truly, the devil is in the details and a lot of times we can seek and receive from our truest friends the support we need by simply stating what we feel in response to our experience. And it is what we feel about the details that are invariably more significant anyway. Learning to account for our emotions—the good and the bad of them— on our own, fortifies us to learn and grow in ways specific to our maturity as individuals. Bringing us closer to being that exquisite woman, ready for his exquisite love. It's only just after sunrise and there's still time.

—Carol Blades

CHAPTER 11

Finding Black Love

First and foremost, DO YOU LOVE YOURSELF?? Ladies...please take a few minutes and ponder that one. This is serious we are talking about your life and possibly a lifetime.

The extent that you love yourself is the extent you'll be able to give love, and find it in return.

Looking for Black Love...it all starts with YOU. You are the core of it all. Don't expect to love and build with the next person if you don't love yourself. It's not going to happen! Find your innermost self before you look for a man.

Love yourself for being who you are, doing what you do, saying what you say, thinking what you think, and feeling what you feel. When you do, you make space to be, do, think, feel, express and accept yourself as you are.

Once you love yourself fully you will attract and recognize true pure love around yon Once you find the lover you long for and deserve, you will rise and shine to new levels in your life. Love is a journey with an endless road...

Love your skin color, love your curves, love your kinky hair, and love all the wonderful features that make you the Black woman you are. Love yourself NOW! Don't wait until you lose the weight, or get money, or find a better job, or find a man. It starts now with YOU. That's the bottom line!

If you invest time, patience, communication and love in "me" then the chances of a successful "we" increase. Keep in mind that an investment in "self is an investment in all of your relationships so this applies for all areas in your life.

I believe that loving yourself is the greatest love of all and we all need to love ourselves to have a balanced life. Don't think that's being selfish...it's not! It's simply called self-love. You will be amazed how your attitude and love for self will change your life and you will begin to receive greatness on different aspects in life. Trust me!

Be yourself... truthfully Accept yourself... gratefully
Value yourself... completely
Treat yourself... generously Balance yourself... harmoniously
Bless yourself... abundantly
Trust yourself... confidently

Empower yourself... prayerfully
Give yourself... enthusiastically Express yourself... radiantly Honor yourself... purposefully Love yourself... wholeheartedly
—Author Unknown

If you love yourself, have time, patience and understanding. You're ready to take on anything that comes into your life. It may not happen overnight and don't expect it to, but it will happen and once it does the rest will follow.

In the book The Art of Loving, it describes love as an art that requires patience, confidence, discipline, concentration, faith and practice daily.

So as you can see this is not a change for the moment kind of thing...it's a habit that has to become part of your daily life. You may think that all of this is bullshit and you feel that you know all of this already. Most of us know of it.. .but there is a difference with knowing and doing. If you know it...apply it and you will see the changes.

Keeping things real...find yourself before you look for a man. Don't sit around waiting for Mr. Right to come along and sweep you off your feet. You may end up alone for a long time if you do so. This is not a fairytale or a soap opera this is real life in the real world. Be realistic about the situation and don't lie to yourself...you'11 only end up with disappointment. There's a difference between LOVE and LUST. Lust is a very powerful, very intense feeling of physical attraction toward another person. Lust is mainly sexual in nature—the attraction is superficial based on instant chemistry rather than genuine caring. Usually we lust after people we do not know well, people we still feel comfortable fantasizing about. It is very common for people to confuse lust for love. So be aware of what it is you feel and don't get caught up in lust.

There's no easy way to love a Black man. And for something that may come around once in a lifetime it shouldn't be easy. This takes time, and shouldn't be rushed. Who you share yourself with is important and you should take your time and enter the relationship with your eyes wide open. Approach love very slowly, clearheaded, and careful. People use the word LOVE too loosely and fall in LOVE too easily. Look at the many different settings and situations you may find yourself in when one is in a relationship. Be honest about who you are, your expectations and know your wants and desires. You want to know that who you are and what you feel can survive in a relationship.

Taking on the wonderful venture of loving a black man is serious business but it is well worth it. What you put in and what you'll discover will be MAGICAL. Such love will require the foundation of integrity, communication, understanding, truthfulness, and a want for unity. A meaningful relationship needs time to grow, so again...take your time.

It may be hard on him to give himself to you at first. We have to understand with all the stereotypes that has been put on Black women (unappreciative, uneducated, disrespectful, ignorant, lazy, manipulating, selfish, money hungry and the list goes on and on). That being said...it may take a while for him to build enough trust in you, so please have patience, lots of it. I'm truly sorry that some men may feel that way about us. It's unfortunate that they have come across some Black women who have made them feel that way. But ladies, please try to have a positive outlook and show him that we are different. I do get offended when people say that all Black women do this and do that. Not all Black women embody the numerous stereotypes mentioned. But at the same time, ladies we have to stop ourselves from doing the same thing to our Black men. Too often I hear a Black woman say "all niggas are trifling" or "no good" etc... That's not true. And please let us stop using "niggas" as a reference to BLACK PEOPLE. As much as that word is used, let's not forget where it came from. It's time for us to stop stereotyping our Black men and Black women and LOVE one another and set the example for our children.

When you negatively stereotype ALL or some Black men, you run the risk of overlooking the person that does meet your criteria and your chance at true love and greatness. Look deeper than the surface... yes he may look good but he could end up being a real ass.

Always keep in mind The Laws of Attraction...if you keep saying there's no good Black men...all you will attract is just that! You get what you think about, whether wanted or unwanted. Society wants it this way...they want us to hate on each other and destroy the power that Black people exude and we have let it happen for too long. Love yourself as an individual and show love to your people.

Leave all the "I don't need a man" "I can do bad all by myself bull crap alone. We all know this is not what you desire. If it were, you wouldn't be reading "Looking for Black Love". What you should be saying is "I will be with a great man" "I want a man to share and build with me" and so forth. Make sure he sees your values and feels YOU and what you're about. Make him rethink his so-called notion of the Black woman. Go the extra mile but always stay true to yourself.

I'm not saying that any Black Man is deserving of your love...yes be careful on who you choose. Not all are worthy of being with a Black woman. This is why I have to stress the advice, LEARN YOUR MAN. Who he is, his values, what he's been through, his wants out of life, what he strives for, just learn who he is and welcome what he lays out to you. Take the time and learn everything that makes him the Black man that he is and possibly the man that you want. Not because you find that he displays certain qualities make him the right one for you. Sure enough we all know that when a Black man walks into a room, everyone notices. A Black man's power is intoxicating, but please don't let that be the main thing you look for. There's so much more to a Black man than his beautiful chocolate skin...if you look at them deep down you will see their mind, their strength, their sharpness, how they carry' the burdens of this world gracefully and without complaint and so much more and that to me is what is so captivating of the Black man.

The first thing you must understand, you've got to figure him out. In learning what he's all about, don't forget to show him what you're about. Don't be afraid to explore him pound for pound. DON'T HOLD BACK!! No lies, no deceit, not secrets. Just be YOU in your full essence. If you hold back...you may end up losing out on the greatest thing of all "LOVE".

Once you learn what he's about, take time to weigh out what you can offer. Are you able to handle who he is without trying to change him? Too often I a hear woman, "Oh he's like this and like that" but I can change that. NO! NO! NO! Please, DON'T DO THAT! You must want to be with someone for whom they are.. .not what you think you can mold them to be. If you feel the need to change the person that you are with, then you don't need to be with that person. He's not the one. But if he is., .then see if he's someone you can't live without. If you feel in all of your being that you can't live without him make sure you shower him with sweetness. But never let him mistake your kindness for weakness. Don't let past relationships get in the way of what you want and need. When you first get together enjoy the moments shared and please, please don't comment on it, don't discuss it with your friends, don't have long conversations with your relatives about your new man. Learn him on your own. Communication is very important in any and all relationships.

Okay! We all think we know how to communicate, but I also know that one may feel interrogated when they get into a discussion. So it's important that we know how, when, and what to communicate. If you find that your relationship is fulfilling, but have small issues, keep working at them. Keep talking it out, and stay honest and open. We all have issues to work through and, as a result, experience relationship struggles. We can work it out, but only if we keep working at it and finding a solution. If you're always complaining and don't have a way to solve what's at hand than you enter a vicious circle that may cause your union to end. "It's because of you I'm like this...I said that because you did this...and it's because of you...you...you...that this, this and that is happening". PLEASE! Let's stop the bullshit. You can't blame the other person for all the wrong doings. YOU are in control of yourself and your emotion. If you know yourself you will know how to control what it is you feel either by anger, or hurt. It's easy to blame the next person...be accountable for your wrong doings and watch how you say things. At time it could also be that you need to change some of your ways...try it sometimes, try to change something about yourself and see how he will react to it. I've learned that at times we as women tend to be set in our ways and we don't leave room to think differently. Always remember that you teach your man to treat you in the way you are with him...in the way you respond.

Black men base much of their self-esteem on their performance. But their deeper selves, their motivations, self-image, and fears are often hidden in a private world that they can't, or won't share with their partners. Give him time to process his emotions and understand yours. Trust is so important in any relationship...trust is built over time and by one's actions. I know it takes a lot for some to trust but again...if you took the time to learn your man you would understand why it's hard for him to trust. It's now for you to show your patience and have great understanding. Don't think it's YOU...most of the time it's not...it's all the broken promises of the past that comes into play. Time ladies...time.

When you're in a relationship, list what you appreciate out of him and let him know. You must be appreciative of the little things he tries to do and make sure you do the little things in return. Let him know your word is bond and that he can confide in you. And in return he won't have to hide things from you because he will know that no matter what...you're there. Support him in his decision and be a friend to his foe. Be understanding of what's at hand and don't demand. When he makes a mistake don't say I told you so. Be understanding, not demanding. Work with him, not against him. He has to fight enough in the outside world. Even when they do everything right and play by the book they still don't get the respect they deserve and that's hard to deal with daily. Show him your pride, stand by his side and he will give his all to you.

Make your home happy, let it be his sanctuary where he can unwind and be free. Be his sunshine and keep him warm. Let him come to his comfort zone and run to the one that he knows love him. The last thing he wants is to come home to nags and complaints. A man wants to know that once he enters his home he can relax and leave all the stress of the outside world...outside. Would you enjoy coming home to someone that from the moment your walk into a room they are full of complaints and so forth? NO!! Well neither does he.

In making your home happy, other things come into play. Yes, you want to keep a clean house, but you also want to keep yourself together. Remember to be sexy without a doubt and look good when he gets home. Not only for him...but for you as well. You will feel better about yourself and that will reflect in other areas. So never forget, don't let yourself go, don't forget about you. Men are more visual...it has nothing to do with them being shallow... that's just how it is... so make it exciting for him. I'm not saying to be in lingerie every day when he comes home, but surely you can clean up well and fix yourself a bit to make it more pleasing to the eye. Would you like seeing your man not well groomed in a T-shirt, shorts and flip-flops every day? I know I don't...I been there and after a while there was nothing exciting about it.

Cook nice meals and be attentive to his needs...run his shower and follow it by a full body massage. Take care of your man and show him how much you appreciate him. In doing so he will feel your love and you will get all the love you deserve in return.

Keep love exciting and new. The bedroom should not be the only place you make love. Spice it up every now and then and don't forget that making love doesn't always consist of long slow lovemaking. A fuck here and there doesn't mean that he doesn't love you because he's not lying up with you for hours on end. A quickie is fun...be spontaneous...let loose. Explore other ways in being intimate. Keep finding new ways to make him smile. When he smiles...you will smile, too. When you love your man, love him all the way down. Don't hold back. You only end up missing out.

Give him what he needs to feel...if you don't I guarantee that someone else will. Yes, he may be content with what you give him and yes, he may stay but it will be for the wrong reasons. Be all that you can be. And a wonderful Black man is what you'll get.

Ok...who am I to say this to you? I am a black woman that has wanted to find love. In my past relationships, I had to really look at what was at hand and the hardest thing was being honest with myself on who I was and what I really wanted. I got tired of cheating myself out of greatness and pretending that life was great. I finally learned to love myself for who I was and laid out what it was I could offer a man. I was single for over 5 years before I met the love of my life. Finding "THE ONE" is the most amazing feeling ever. And you can trust that it comes in the strangest places and when you least expect it. I for one am very fortunate to have found "THE ONE". He's my king and I will always treat him as such. It took a long time before he came into my world. But from the first moment we met I knew I had found him. It's humanly impossible to describe the feeling it brings. Elevation of the heart and mind is the most beautiful thing one can ever experience.

We have built a strong foundation with communication, understanding, honesty, a great friendship and so much more...it's out there ladies. Black men are out there and when you find him...love your man and show him how much he is appreciated in every way. By doing so you will obtain your heart's desire.

—Michelle King

CHAPTER 12

Sistahs, Let's Wake Up

I was sitting in the make-up chair as Landis prepared my face for camera, lights, and action. Landis happens to be one of Chicago's premier make-up artists. I was really looking forward to my first "facelift" in his chair. He was transitioning me from the savvy but hurried-looking professional sistah to television talk show guest. Landis and I made seemingly idle conversation for a few moments as he applied my powders, shadows and liners when I realized we had some mutual acquaintances. Before I knew it, we were on the subjects of; what Black women say they want from Black men, what they get and why. Landis shared, "Women get exactly what they ask for based on the standards of today's Black woman." What he didn't realize was I'd be in full agreement. Our conversation became the story of a beautiful love affair gone counterfeit.

I don't expect to be applauded for what I am about to share. I didn't create it. But I did contribute, and it is time we, as Black women, begin to look at the issue of the downward spiral of Black male/female relationships. We must collectively take the lead in a paradigm shift that must occur before healing. Too few of us [Black women] really want to deal with the muddled state of the Black male/female dynamic and typically when I share my views about this subject my sistahs get very defensive, which is often our reaction when discussing this same issue with our men. Many sistahs believe I set Black women back 50 years when I speak on this subject; however, this has never been my intent. I am simply one Black woman whose paradigm shifted. I desire that our relationships heal and once again become whole. Why not take some responsibility?

I won't bore you with any details of slavery and Its devastating effects on the Black male/female psyche. We know this story all too well. But, I will share that it appears to me that we have dropped the "relational ball". We've replaced our intelligent Black brother, friend, confidante, protector; provider, husband and lover—yes our Black lion—for the trappings of success, money and power. When did we drop the ball? Well, I contend when we entered Corporate America! The 'drop' was not a flagrant attempt to devalue Black men, however, a subtle shift in our values and family structure placated often by an ever-changing American economic climate.

During the late 50's and throughout the 60's, many Black men were struggling and making it happen in factory and plant jobs throughout the United States. Black men were seeking out a good life for themselves and their families. These same men once afforded opportunities moved into what we now call "blue collar" positions with the US Postal Service and other city and government jobs. We were building our middle class—finally. Some of these men were even able to make it into white-collar positions as foremen and managers. But when the factories and plants began to close their doors and layoffs were announced, our men moved from gainful employment to joblessness. Black women - the strong sistahs we've always been—entered the marketplace to assist our men in supporting the family. We were the 'insurance' policy, if you will. Never looking at this as a power move, but a helpmeet move. During those lean times we entered the workforce until our men found gainful employment. It was always done in love--for love and survival of the family.

I know Black women have traditionally worked. We've cleaned home—not always our own, cooked meals—not always for ourselves or our families, washed clothes and took care of children—not just our own. We also nurtured and loved our men and families. It was truly a love affair. We supported our husbands and brothers. We stood by their sides and encouraged them to greatness. It was okay to cook his meal and warm his sheets at night. It was okay to push him higher. It wasn't slave labor; it was our love labor. We didn't have to do it. We did it seasoned in our struggle. We were in love. We knew together we could overcome any obstacle, and our children watched as we navigated through rough waters as a cohesive unit— not separate but equal.

Nevertheless, with the women's revolution well underway, a convoluted economic shift emerged in 1970. A great white wave flooded into the homes of Black America, which I believe moved our men from pillars of provider and strength in our communities to the lines of despair, abandonment and unemployment. With this came what I call the age of "entrapment" for Black women. We went to college; we got jobs and became secretaries and administrative assistants. We graduated from college; got better jobs, promotions and raises. Pivotally, we were now accepted in the corporate workplace above our men, a strategic spiritual and economic tool used, which, presently, many of us are still blinded by this. We were given positions that once belonged to our husbands and brothers. We were accepted. We became his [our brothers'] "boss". We had it goin' on and everybody knew it. "I am woman. Hear me roar" was chanted from the mouths of women, both Black and White, but whose song was it really? Culturally speaking, it is the male lion that roars—struts. I know some of us won't get that.

As we began to bring home the bacon, we also began to view our husbands, brothers and male acquaintances differently. He was now becoming a thorn in our side; he was keeping us down. We were now able to afford upscale lunches at the finest restaurants in downtown USA and designer clothing adorned our backs. The feminist movement, which was never our movement said, "We had rights. We were entitled." We watched as the "Boss" bought presents for his wife during lunch—because he was dating the secretary. We watched as the "Boss" drove his BMW and Mercedes into the workplace and we, the nurturers and lovers of our men, homes and families began to covet this lifestyle. Discontent entered our unions like a gentle breeze.

Armed with degrees, corporate power and money we brought it "correct" to our men: "Either get a job or a better job. Make some money or get out! Why can't you afford roses—which I once grew in my garden, but today I have little time for? Why don't we buy a car like the "Boss"? Why can't we wear more designer labels like the "Boss"? Why can't we buy a bigger house like the "Boss"? I can do this by myself! I don't need you! You are holding me back!' What happened?

We told our men they were no longer needed and expected them to stay. We told them to get out, but we closed the open door. We told them their money wasn't enough, but we wanted them to buy our dinner. We told him his house was too small and apartment was too shabby—so we bought bigger ones his salary could not afford. We told him he didn't measure up to our "Boss", so we didn't take him to the corporate functions. We told him his good simply wasn't good enough. We stopped loving, inspiring, building, motivating—we stopped caring. Not only did we tell him, we showed him by bringing in the big dollars and falling in love with the "Boss".

To make matters sweeter [for Black women] Congress passed an important law in 1975. This law had far reaching implications for the Black Family. That would be the equal Credit Opportunity Act, which said, among other things that banks could no longer ignore a sistah's income when determining whether the family earned enough money to qualify for a mortgage. So we bought even bigger houses. Doesn't sound too earth shattering and the question here is not if the Act was needed, however, I submit this Act opened the door for us sistahs to take our money, buy our house and run when it didn't make sense. We began to look at our positions as mother, wife, daughter and sister as menial labor. These were 'positions' relegated to poor and uneducated woman. Now, one generation later and what a mess. We no longer wanted to be like our mothers keeping the house, cooking, loving our men and our children. That job was for suckers. The world had so much more to offer. Or so we thought.

Today we've kicked brothers completely to the curb. Sorry brothers catch up if you can. I see a bus coming. We have and plan children whom we believe we can and should raise alone. What? We buy and build our own homes with no intention of a brother ever living there, because it's mine. We manage over brothers in our positions as vice president and CFO—catch up if you can now. We lease our Lexus and Jaguar and we will not date a brother who doesn't own property. We have more disposable income since entering the workforce and climbing the corporate ladder, however we're spending more trying to keep up with the "Boss". We raise our children in daycare centers and with home care providers with little or no guilt. We nurture less and love less. Then we ask why a brother doesn't want to open a car door. We wonder why the brother doesn't want to pay the mortgage. We wonder why he wants to go 'Dutch'. We wonder why he dates White women. We wonder why he doesn't want to serve our God and enter our churches. Who is our God anyway? We wonder why our brother doesn't want to talk anymore. We wonder why there exists a disconnection between Black men and women. Are we really that blind? Sistahs, we've usurped from our men their role as Black men. We've taken from our men their purpose and place in our lives; however, as Landis so fondly shared, 'We still want to hold brothers accountable to the standards of yesteryear.' I tend to agree with brothers who say, 'Enough is enough'. Black women, we can't have what our double mind speaks because we're tearing brothers down! Just like the crack of "Boss" whip.

I know we are not going to stop working sistahs! This is not what I suggest. Many of us have careers we love and are in no position to leave Corporate America, even if we wanted to. Many of us hold positions, which will help change and shape the world. I certainly do not advocate throwing in the towel on higher education for Black women. But I challenge us sistahs to pause for a moment and contemplate what our actions and words are saying to Black men and where they've gotten us. Yes, I know we are educated and powerful Black women who can verbally spar and out think and run companies with the best of them. We do it all day in Corporate America, but why bring it home? I challenge us sistahs to ask ourselves some questions: When did I stop offering my labor of love to my Black man? When did the Black man become my enemy? Can I take responsibility for what I've created? When did I start believing the lie that my worth status and success should be measured by the dollars we make? Who told me his Buick was whack and Corporate America is all that? When did our homes change from his castle of peace to a den of thieves?

Let's travel back to a time when 'bringing home the bacon and frying it up in a pan' wasn't our dream. That was never our story. We have our media induced ethics to thank for that. You see, I remember watching nana give papa a wet kiss when he returned home from a hard day's work. I remember smelling baked chicken, greens and cornbread coming from the homes, which line Carpenter Street, as mothers, sisters and daughters prepared dinner for their husbands, sons and brothers. These Black men were our champions and heroes. I remember when our homes were safety zones and a place of refuge, protection—comfort for Black men. The walls were fortified with love, peace, patience and kindness. The enemy could not penetrate. I remember a day when Black was beautiful on a brother. I remember a day when I'd get on the bus and say hello to the brother driving the bus—because he looked like me—and I'd greet the brother I sat next to. I remember a day when I'd walk into the grocery store and the Black man behind the counter was my brother—he was my uncle, father—he'd give me the best cut of meat. I'd thank him and ask about his family and day. I'd smile as he asked about my father. What a love story! Brother Landis, all I can say is I remember!
—Serene Bridgett Hollingsworth

Serene Bridgett Hollingsworth is by God's grace a child of the living God, daughter sister, mother of four girls and CEO/Publisher and Editorial director of Bahiyah Woman Magazine (BWM) www.BWMMag.com— the magazine empowering the spiritually conscious professional Black man and woman. She currently resides in Chicago, Illinois with her family.

Understanding

The whole race is suffering because of a hunger that permeates every aspect of life. Our phenomenal women who have re-defined excellence in America can't even express their full potential because it's hard to focus, accomplish, and achieve when you are starving. Women's hearts are undernourished, under-nurtured, and under assault. How can you build your greatest structures, your greatest establishments, and your greatest societies when you don't have someone to rejuvenate your life giving energy? And what energy on the planet has proven to be greater than love?

We men are not doing a good job of providing our women with her most basic need—Love and Support. We have left her hungry, cold, and without shelter. Almost all our problems as a race can be traced back to the fact that we aren't loving our women enough, we aren't working hard enough to sustain our love and relationships, and we aren't doing enough to build alongside our women in a way that's going to enrich and fulfill our children.

Men have dropped the ball and until we pick it up, get a game plan and utilize teamwork, Black men and Blackwomen will remain firmly behind the 8-ball as a societal force on this planet.

Women you can ill-afford to sit by, holding your breath, waiting for the Black man to get his shit together. You need to start coaching him, training him, redirecting his focus and attention away from Bling Bling back towards surviving, flourishing, achieving greatness together—Black man, Black woman, and child, side by side the way it was always meant to be. This is the greatest path to Power for Blackwomen facing today's challenges. Until that cohesive union can; be accomplished, it is paramount to Our survival that you continue to survive and flourish, using Supreme strength and intelligence; From God To Earth.

Chapter 13

A Real Conversation Between God and Earth

This chapter is the real communication between a man and a woman; a god and an earth. These e-mails are builds between two intelligent people who have 'knowledge of self. They have studied 'The Book of Life', which is the 120° lessons taught by The Nation of Gods and Earths; commonly known as The Five Percenters.

In the Nation, Blackman are called Gods and Blackwomen are called Earths; for they are both the physical manifestation of the divine. Within these e-mails you can find the evolution of this book. Plus, you witness two people try to build an understanding between themselves, while trying to find some answers to better help women and their various circumstances.

A few terms used in these e-mails may be unfamiliar like:

Math - it's a language used by Gods and Earths, which give each numeral a meaning.

Alphabets - is a dialect used by Gods and Earths, which gives each alphabet a meaning.

Parliament - is a gathering of Gods and Earths every last Sunday of the month, that takes place across the country and a few places abroad.

All Being Born To (A,B.B.T.) - is the summation of math to arrive at a higher meaning.

Seeds and Stars - the children.

Wisdom - the woman.

Sun - the men.

I hope this witnessing of our private builds (positive communication), never intended for print give the readers; especially the women a glimpse at the awesome power 'knowledge of self' can provide.

Peace Earth, I come in the divine name of Power and I have had knowledge of self, knowledge power years.

Been trapped in the belly just as long, but extreme hardship doesn't always just create pain - sometimes it creates positivity. I have become a student of life, a teacher of young minds, and an accomplished author.
I found your 'Vanilla is Black' both entertaining and enlightening. I am also attracted to a clean, holistic lifestyle.
I was impressed with you and felt a pull towards your thoughts and unique background.
Plus I do ceramics too :)

Peace God - I be the Earth and have had KOS for almost knowledge wisdom rotations. I appreciate your kind words. It was a short piece but was hard for me to put myself out there and I'm thankful that it affected folks in the way that it did. What kind of ceramic work do you do and what exactly about holistic living are you drawn to? Peace on Wisdom Born

Peace Earth, I wanted to elaborate on why I reached out, yesterday i was moving fast and my build was brief.
Like I said I was impressed with the words and credentials. I am very interested in Holistic living and eating, especially for women from a women's perspective. I am the author of 5 books including 'Gods Earths, and 85er's' and 'Consequences of Oppression'. I'm working on a 'Consequences of Oppression' part 2 and could use your knowledge and insight to try and combat our people's dangerous diets in a chapter i named 'Dying to Eat'.
Plus, you seem to have that entrepreneurial spirit and I'm very focused in those areas. I expect to re-entry to the free cipher this year and one of my goals is to create a positive oasis called' True Nature Retreat", where people can go and heal their bodies and nourish their minds, while finding solace away from the stress and strains of the city. Sound like that's up your alley, right?
In short, beautiful, wise Queen I think our rotation could be powerful and our build divine.

Peace God - That sounds like a beautiful plan to make manifest. I'd be interested in adding on to a project yet I should be upfront and also say that I am a mother of three, run and operate a community farm, lead a community garden and add on to collaborative writing projects across the wilderness... that being said I have spread myself thin and am making intentional efforts to work toward better time management. I have the genetic trait of "obligatory service" meaning I feel like I owe the world something., .everything, and so while the idealist in self hears your request and says,"sign me up", my rational mind (that is the secondary voice) says " can you give the proper attention to a project like that?". So while you are making your plan manifest, what I would offer to you is some free consultation, but I can't commit to a partnership or an emotional, intellectual, physical investment. U see me? When do you re-enter the free cipher and where will you be located? Earth-centered living is my life, because I am the Earth, and even before I had knowledge of self as the Earth I was drawn to all things related to the Earth, so the knowledge was epiphanic for me. and so you knowledge... I am humbled by your request as I would say that there are many sisters across the wilderness that have credentials far greater than mine. Peace on Understanding Knowledge

Peace Earth, UR e-mail is like refined, refreshing water. I just came from a cipher - the first last Sunday of the decade. I built on entrepreneurship, made my library available and told a God how righteous it felt to have a true and living Earth greet me with Peace God. I never built with a Earth that already had KOS.
can I ask out of respect - do u have a God? Even though I'm not in search of a mental, emotional, or physical
commitment :), I want to be respectful. Plus, I wanted to know before I asked permission to call u V. Queen :) Your Vanilla Parfait left such a tasty impression on me.
Queen I recognize u have a tremendously full plate, especially raising 3 precious seeds. My goal isn't to take ur time and energy, but to give u some of mine. Maybe I could more beautify ur world with my ceramics and words. And having u to consult with, build with, or just get to know, i believe will broaden my perspectives and understanding, and better my writing. Already
I feel like your Earthly wisdom and presence could be my muse.
My oasis/center idea is further in the future, my immediate goals is open my Royal Books and Tees stores, continue publishing,

and do a documentary on our Nation based on my book 'Gods, Earths and 85er's'. Have u ever read any of my books? Can I send u 'Consequences of Oppression'?
I should be free this year and I have plans to open my first store in Orlando, FL area, but Denver could be next:)
Queen I would like to get to know U, on ur terms - at ur pace. I know U R very special with a very special and busy Cipher – I understand and would not be interested if I didn't think I could add - not subtract.
My Chocolate is attracted to ur Vanilla in so many ways other than physical - and I think that's a great place to start. Don't You?
Peace

Peace God. So um...that was a lot of innerG in that last communiqué. I had to take a minute to digest it. Let's slow up a bit 1) I'm not currently committed, yet there are a few suitors (nothing physical). 2) I am swift and changeable and knowledge that about myself 3) Have had some unsavory long distance experiences and 4) I don't even knowledge you. So, why don't you tell me a story, *Your* story. I'm most intrigued. Peace on Wisdom.

Peace,
O.K. I understand - strictly consultation :)
So, what u know about the Lymph System and Toxemia?
I'm trying to enlighten more people, especially Blackwomen about the need to keep their Lymph System clean and healthy to prevent disease and illness. Also the advantages of monodieting and eating less animal products - which we know contributes the most toxins. I just stopped eating chicken and cheese to end all animal products - except I'm undecided about fish, what's ur opinion on fish? and I decided this new book will be called 'AND GOD CREATED WOMEN, But Men Created These Fucked-up Conditions' U Like ?   And I apologize if earlier I was too fast and forward! THANKS
Much Respect and Peace

Peace God - FYI, I wasn't avoiding you, it's just that internet time is limited for me and this is a heavy planning time of year for a vegetable farmer (me), but to offer some clarity I am most def NOT looking for any additional suitors, especially ones whom I have not met in the physical and who clearly have romanticized the idea. Please brother, let's keep it business. You can decide if you are attracted to a woman when you meet her and can do the knowledge to her mannerisms and ways and actions. And I would challenge your title as I am not a feminist but a womanist and see that most so-called patriarchal ideas are eurocentric more than they are patriarchal. I agree lymph is the key to a woman's optimal health. My opinion on fish is that if our planet were running at optimal health than it would be wise to eat fresh water fish, however our waters are polluted and our fish are bred and farmed so I would say that one should forego the fish unless they could ensure that wild and clean (unlikely in the wilderness of north america.) If its fish oil that you are advocating than I would suggest flax, primrose, and coconut oil as an alternative. Peace

Peace Earth, how r u? Is this cold damaging the crops? Farming sounds hard, but rewarding. So is there a big cipher in Denver? who do u build with - u seem very sharp ! And how do u see the debate over whether the woman is Earth or Goddess?
I don't get bent out of shape about her being called Goddess, but because Goddess would mean she can create everything in existence -1 disagree. Even though we both have the Seven elements that created everything in the Universe: Proton,
Neutron, Electron, Strong Force, Weak Force, Gravity, and Electromagnetism - Man has both X and Y chromosome,
She has 2 X chromosomes - so scientifically Man could create Woman, born-u-truth Woman can't create MAN.
What's UR understanding?

Peace Allah -
The cipher here is small and even fewer have actually knowledged 120. I studied with brothers here as well as long distance and my journey thru 120 had some disconnects and I did have to renew my history a few times. I have built with people on either side of that argument and I had to draw it up for myself in the end. For me there has yet to be a scientific argument to call a woman Goddess. In actuality I would rather call a man Allah than call him God which is a greek word in itself. I see myself as the Earth divine and equal but not God. I have no aspirations to be as I am fulfilled in the complexities of the Earth. I do take issue with brothers who assume- that the Earth is Less than Allah, and have the linear programming that the order of things has some bearing on the quality of things. I am the Earth. Allah came first and I am his compliment, not a limitation, but a compliment, the Earth absorbs and Transforms and is the Home of Islam. Allah is the God of the Universe and The Earth is the Queen of the physical and emotional frequencies within.... u know Macrocosms and Microcosms... He provides the seed of life and she absorbs, carries and nurtures it to bring forth life. They are intrinsically connected. Be Well
Peace on Knowledge Culture

Peace Earth, how R U? U and your positive energy has been a big help. I almost finished chapter Dying to Eat/ Eating to live.
I discussed food combining, the need 4 high water content foods (70%), ridding the body of toxins, proper fruit consumption, Natural Body Cycles 1. Eating and Digestion 2. Absorbtion 3. Elimination. I expand on the need to reduce or eliminate animal products and dairy. Anything u want to add? Why did U become a vegan? How did the change affect U?
What's a proper diet 4 women?   I also changed the title: 'From God To Earth: A Serious Conversation'
Do U like that better? I would like to send U a copy of chapter 4 inspection and insight. I would be surprised if someone
as professional and aloof (at least towards me :)   didn't have a P.O. Box.
Peace and thanks for being there!

Peace,
I became vegan when I was 15, and wavered a bit back to veg when I was negotiating having a meat eater for a partner (my seeds father), and am back to vegan now. I became vegan as I was learning more about nutrition and industrial farming... and to be very honest I was more moved to be vegan as an act of resistance to industrial establishment that for health benefits. I still to this day don't harbor judgment toward folks who eat meat and especially when they are indigenous people eating their indigenous diet... however we live in the wilderness of north america and here we have a choice (even tho many are blind deaf and dumb to the choices). The changes in my body and in my life were dramatic. 1) any bodily function or process that was compromised before I became veg, was amplified after, but the benefit to that is that being able to identify and correct things to put your body back into balance. 2) I was ostracized by my friends and family because here where I live only the Caucasian is veg.... so I had to be really intentional about feeding myself and making sure I was grounded in my reasons and intentions. I'm not easily swayed when I make a decision and make sure that I am educated when discussing my life choices....
I think it would be arrogant for me to speak on what is good for women across the world but I do know that we need to be really careful about phytoestrogens in our food and additional hormones... it is hard to balance the world of hormones in the wilderness of north america...in our water food and medicine and that is one thing that I would say all women need to pay attention to the other thing is managing and balancing our b12 intake... it is a life saver and directly related to our hormones and emotions...
I'd be happy to read whatever you send ...no p.o. box. I'll give you a physical address so long as you don't become a stalker.
;-)
I have a few questions for you.
1)   how do you manage to eat a balanced vegetarian diet in the pen? how can you? are you getting all the nutrients you need?
2)   what are you in for? I was gonna hold off on asking but if we are going to have a business relationship you ought to go ahead and reveal it.
3)   what's your physical degree, how did you receive KOS and how long have you had it? (just being nosy here) Peace on Wisdom Understanding

I appreciate your honesty, and I build that I eventually change your 'wary' to comfort and constructiveness.

I can imagine your schedule is extremely busy, especially raising 3 stars. They sound extremely bright and I'm sure having u 4 a mom is a tremendous asset. I understand the no force policy -1 wasn't able to persuade my son to join the culture, especially from such a distance. Still trying to reach him, sending him 'Rap, Rage and REV.' to stimulate his mental. What do u think of the God's book? Powerful Elevation!

Understanding-culture, huh? If I was a suitor, that would be a perfect degree :)

So how's that going - any suitors convince u to orbit around them exclusively yet?

Do u believe the Earth can only receive the light and energy of one Sun, even if the Sun is capable of shining on to many planets?

The package I sent should arrive soon, looking forward to your honest build - and don't worry about your perceived lack of tact sometimes -1 value Truth and Honesty above all.

I build u and your seeds are very well.

Peace

P.S. Is it true Colorado has some of the best water?

Again in theory the idea that the Earth revolves around 1 Sun suits me, but I've been single and studying a long time... so I have to take in the physical sunlight and study with my brothers...

The God Supreme Understanding is a really knowledgeable brother... and his books are well written and relatable to the youth, good choice...

I look forward to receiving the package. Peace on Knowledge Equality

Peace, I build u r well, tho very busy. That build was peace, u should receive various lights

and continue to nourish your mental to its fullest - especially till U born an understanding with a i ,d strong enough to accept

only his light and energy. Again, this is a unique and long over-due experience, I think will raise my standards :)
physical without mental without culture will feel incomplete.
By now u should have received my most recent build and my first ever build 'Consequences' (born that knowledge-wisdom ago, put in rotation myself culture ago).
Power for me is an attribute and more - a pursuit. That's why I chose Media, It's one of the greatest tools of Power - to be able to influence, teach, spread words, images, info. So I own 7 books, about 100 songs, a few movie scripts and the means to born them. If the devil has all tools of the power, everyone else will always lose. I'm just trying to add more balance.
Media is Power that's not a necessity; like now books are slow. I want to also build on a need (food, clothing, shelter). What's more needed than Water? One day, an All-Natural Life Water, with natural flavoring from organic sources and 1. slightly alkaline, 1. slightly acidic, 1. balanced PH. Provide free PH strips so people can test themselves to find their need, (most people are acidic), alkaline water would increase their health and longevity. I heard Colorado has some of the cleanest and best tasting water in the U.S.   Do you agree?   Maybe that's my reason to come to Colorado and be near one day.
Great Water and Great Wisdom!
Peace Earth, always a pleasure building with you!

Peace God -1 haven't received the package yet...should probably come any day. I suppose the drinking water here is good. We have some natural springs that are lovely for sure.
I'll just say this many brothers in the belly have reached out to build, and sadly many of them can't form proper sentences. Just saying that its nice that you spent your time in solitude like a monk, ever learning ever elevating... born u truth I want to remind you that it's not wise to court a person whom you've never met... so ease up. ;-)
Peace on the Queens Day.

Peace, you are a nerd, lucky for u I like nerds. Dancing Dragons and The Toa of Physics sounds interesting,
your library may be better than mine. Daydream about plants, you are so unique there.
I guess that package got lost somewhere between here and the Rockies. It contained the chapter on health, a copy of my Consequences of Oppression' and a picture of me and some ceramics I done.

Why are u so selective about my comments - am I on punishment for sounding to flirty or courting? :)

Peace Power,
Today's Supreme Math is Wisdom Equality abbt Build and Destroy. Wisdom is wise words ways and actions, what makes a thing wise is that its rooted in factual data (knowledge), this is why wisdom is the bridge. You can't get that clarity (understanding) on the knowledge you receive unless you bridge it with wisdom. Equality is to deal equality (not the same) in all things. Equality is sharing what you can in a way that is appropriate to the cipher you are dealing with. Build is to add on/ Destroy is to remove or take away. I see these this as integrated into each other, some may disagree however I see that whenever you are building you have to-remove obstacle and whenever you are destroying something is always build from it (whether internal or external).
Our interaction is very interesting to me. You are clearly an intelligent brother with quite a bit to offer the world in the way of knowledge wisdom and understanding... however I have been clear that I don't deal with mystery relationships. Our interaction must be intellectual and have connected in that way because we have something we can share in that cipher. It is not uncomfortable for me that you "court' however it's not realistic and I'm not open to it. I may have built some walls around the notion of long distance courting because of experience I have with it. Also to be really frank, it's important to me that folks who court are physically attracted to each other and we have no way of knowing that...so it is a mystery. So, having said all that...I do enjoy building with you... you're not on punishment, but that's why I only answer certain questions that you ask.... we have to build off of what we know in order for it to be wise.
Peace on Wisdom Equality

Peace, Wow! I have never been so intelligently chastised :), born-u-truth it was worth the build. Strong!
I knowledge that Ours is an intellectual interaction, you have made it abundantly clear that I am unsuitable as a suitor :)
Born-u-truth don't I get some liberties from time to time? like playfulness, flirtatious, even comedic?

You have my respect as an Earth, u have my admiration as a mind, so is it so bad if every now and then I just recognize u as a woman? Is my good-natured compliments and flirting an obstacle? (notice I didn't say courting).

I understand my limitations to well and I won't take any fantastical, mystical mental voyages surrounding Us - b.u.t. I will sometimes stray into non- impersonal intellectual building. That's just the charming part of me - tho u clearly don't find it charming. I enjoyed this build, I feel like I was introduced to Ms. Dragon a lil :)

you told me to ease up - OK, b.u.t. you should chill a lil too - it's not that serious. The God isn't your usual desperate soul looking for anyone to fill a void. I just like to smile around a wisdom and I thought I could make u smile -1 guess I over-estimated my power. Peace and I still think your intellect and refinery is a beautiful thing.

P.S. Which title do you think have more attractive powers for all Blackwomen?

'Black World Order: For Women' or ' From God To Earth: A Serious Conversation For Women"

Peace God. Yup, I suppose that was the dragon. ;-) i do think you are funny and witty and even charming. just get caught up in my defenses from time to time. Pardon. I think you should mix the titles. I'll build more on the next day. Peace to the God Power!

Peace, In response to yesterday's build. Wisdom is the detectable manifestation of knowledge also wise ways and actions. Equality is to deal equal, like giving each new build a chance to show and prove based on its own merits.

Abbt - Build is add on, moving forward in a positive manner, to do that you often have to destroy some pre-conceived notions.

That's why the Earth shouldn't receive too much Sun, it burns the soil and makes it difficult for new vegetation to take root. It takes the proper source, the proper amount, at the proper time to repair that soil.

Built on perfection - the right Wisdom building with the right God to Born a more complete cipher

Peace God -I received the package on the last day (wisdom god). Thank you for sending all this! I'm honored. The reflections are nice too... u got some serious guns! I got some reading to do... I suppose I'll put down the Tao of Physics for a few and peruse through all this masterful literature.

by the way... you have no idea what you're getting into tryna enroll me into your life... Once I'm in I'm hard to shake... which is why I put up so much resistance...

Thank you

Peace, I'm glad the Earth is well and progressing. I did miss your builds and energy, good to know it wasn't just me that had u in absence. Of course, life, raising and resting keeps u busy and the God appreciates the time you have and do expend in his direction. Wanted u to see another side of my lit - and truth be told -1 like being nice to the Earth.

always, Power

Peace on Wisdom Power abbt God.

Went to Parliament today... thought of you being steadfast in the belly (don't get any ideas). Just wanted to send you some warm currents.

A lot of my sisters are in crisis right now regarding the men in their lives.... I am not because I have not let any in.... born universal truth I have to wonder if the lesson is to put in work because I don't have any sisters who are "happy" in their relationships. Maybe the lesson is to have the courage to work through it? Maybe the lesson is to see self with the same critical eye that we see our men with? What's your thoughts on this and the day? Peace

Peace,
It bothers me that even Gods and Earths aren't building harmoniously.

I feel Wisdoms need to empower themselves more, it's harder now to rely on God. We just left an era of selfishness and excess and too many brothers didn't come thru with a sense of self, of family and community responsibility, and the respect and love for our women, now things are extremely arduous for many and we no-longer want to work hard, be disciplined, sacrifice and be steadfast in our goals- for self, economics, for relationships.
"Unhappy" by what standards? is our todays more difficult than our yesterdays ?
So do U feel more or less fortunate to not be in a relationship and be going thru the ups and downs?
and do all warm currents come with a warning ? :)
Peace

Peace on Wisdom Born,
The kind of crisis they are dealing with is physical/mental abuse and sever infidelity... what's the real rationale for those things? Warm currents are warm currents... I was just tryna be funny... (damn internet)
I think our Todays are more 'complicated' than our yesterday's... the more we know, the more we know to look for (good and bad) and maybe the more brilliant we are, the more sever the polarity of our "shadows... I mean however great someone appears, their secrets will be that much more dark and harrowing... it may not be truth, just me pondering the fuckery of humanity...
I know some amazing people... and the above statement seems true enough. I don't have an issue with people being as fucked up as they are amazing, I would just ask that everyone be honest about who they are...
In regards to whether or not I feel more or less fortunate to be 'without a life partner... it would depend on the day. when my sisters are calling me in tears/rage/pain I feel grateful to be without. On other days when I let my mind wander outside of dutiful obligation and the day's work, I might find some solace in a daydream about the Sun...
I dunno. I'm open to new adventures, but I don't know if I can promise "forever" to anyone... that seems unrealistic.
You have thoughts on that?
Peace

This concludes the conversation from God to Earth as manifested by me, Pen Black.

It is my sincerest wish that this book help empower women; especially Blackwomen in ways that will help them fulfill their inherit greatness. I sincerely wish that this book uplift your spirits and make whatever trials you face more surmountable and your triumphs more enjoyable. I also hope this ode to your unique greatness help you realize your goals and realize your accomplishments more fully.

Thank you for allowing our nation to rest on your shoulders for so long.

Peace, Pen Black

When God Made Women

Phenomenal You,
In all your hues,
If the world don't know, then surely I do.
You opened our eyes, eons ago,
and taught Us sciences,
that started our growth.
When you and our lands,
were pillaged and raped,
you fought beside Us in battle,
when needed - planned our escape.
When we were dragged to these shores,
and taught to hate our Black,
what kept Us strong was your love,
and the strength of your back.
So if we forget to tell you,
I apologize for them all,
when God made women of color,
he blessed the whole wide world.